Your *Clinics* subscription ju~~st~~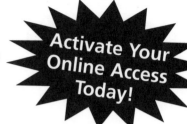

☑ **W9-ABB-105**

You can now access the FULL TEXT of this publication online at no additional cost! Activate your online subscription today and receive...

- Full text of all issues from 2002 to the present
- Photographs, tables, illustrations, and references
- Comprehensive search capabilities
- Links to MEDLINE and Elsevier journals

Activate Your Online Access Today!

Plus, you can also sign up for E-alerts of upcoming issues or articles that interest you, and take advantage of exclusive access to bonus features!

To activate your individual online subscription:

1. Visit our website at www.TheClinics.com.

2. Click on "Register" at the top of the page, and follow the instructions.

3. To activate your account, you will need your subscriber account number, which you can find on your mailing label (note: the number of digits in your subscriber account number varies from six to ten digits). See the sample below where the subscriber account number has been circled.

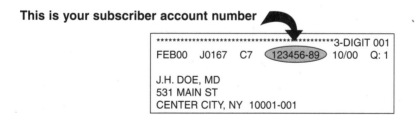

This is your subscriber account number

```
**********************************************3-DIGIT 001
FEB00   J0167   C7   (123456-89)   10/00   Q: 1

J.H. DOE, MD
531 MAIN ST
CENTER CITY, NY  10001-001
```

4. That's it! Your online access to the most trusted source for clinical reviews is now available.

theclinics.com

ELSEVIER

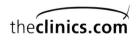

HAND CLINICS

Brachial Plexus Injuries in Adults

GUEST EDITORS
Allen T. Bishop, MD,
Robert J. Spinner, MD,
Alexander Y. Shin, MD

February 2005 • Volume 21 • Number 1

SAUNDERS

An Imprint of Elsevier, Inc.
PHILADELPHIA   LONDON   TORONTO   MONTREAL   SYDNEY   TOKYO

W.B. SAUNDERS COMPANY

A Division of Elsevier Inc.

The Curtis Center • Independence Square West • Philadelphia, Pennsylvania 19106

http://www.theclinics.com

HAND CLINICS	**Volume 21, Number 1**
February 2005	**ISSN 0749-0712**
Editor: Debora Dellapena	**ISBN 1-4160-2660-6**

The ideas and opinions expressed in *Hand Clinics* do not necessarily reflect those of the Publisher. The Publisher does not assume any responsibility for any injury and/or damage to persons or property arising out of or related to any use of the material contained in this periodical. The reader is advised to check the appropriate medical literature and the product information provided by the manufacturer of each drug to be administered to verify the dosage, the method and duration of administration, or contraindications. It is the responsibility of the treating physician or other health care professional, relying on independent experience and knowledge of the patient, to determine drug dosages and the best treatment for the patient. Mention of any product in this issue should not be construed as endorsement by the contributors, editors, or the Publisher of the product or manufacturers' claims.

Hand Clinics (ISSN 0749-0712) is published quarterly by the W.B. Saunders Company. Corporate and Editorial Offices: The Curtis Center, Independence Square West, Philadelphia, PA 19106-3399. Accounting and Circulation Offices: 6277 Sea Harbor Drive, Orlando, FL 32887-4800. Periodicals postage paid at Orlando, FL 32862, and additional mailing offices. Subscription price is $205.00 per year (U.S. individuals), $319.00 per year (U.S. institutions), $103.00 per year (US students), $236.00 per year (Canadian individuals), $355.00 per year (Canadian institutions), $130.00 (Canadian students), $260.00 per year (international individuals), $355.00 per year (international institutions), and $130.00 per year (international students). Foreign air speed delivery is included in all *Clinics* subscription prices. All prices are subject to change without notice. POSTMASTER: Send address changes to *Hand Clinics*, W.B. Saunders Company, Periodicals Fulfillment, Orlando, FL 32887-4800. **Customer Service: 1-800-654-2452 (US). From outside the US, call 1-407-345-4000. E-mail: hhspcs@harcourt.com.**

Reprints. For copies of 100 or more, of articles in this publication, please contact the Commercial Rights Department, Elsevier Inc., 360 Park Avenue South, New York, NY 10010-1710. Tel: (212) 633-3813, Fax: (212) 462-1935, e-mail: reprints@elsevier.com

Hand Clinics is covered in *Index Medicus, Current Contents/Clinical Medicine, EMBASE/Excerpta Medica,* and *ISI/BIOMED.*

Printed in the United States of America.

GUEST EDITORS

ALLEN T. BISHOP, MD, Professor of Orthopedic Surgery, Mayo Medical School; Chair, Division of Hand Surgery, Department of Orthopedic Surgery, Mayo Clinic, Rochester, Minnesota

ROBERT J. SPINNER, MD, Associate Professor, Departments of Neurologic Surgery, Orthopedics, and Anatomy, Mayo Clinic School of Medicine, Rochester, Minnesota

ALEXANDER Y. SHIN, MD, Associate Professor of Orthopedic Surgery, Orthopedic Hand and Microvascular Surgery, Mayo Medical School, Rochester, Minnesota

CONTRIBUTORS

KIMBERLY K. AMRAMI, MD, Consultant in Radiology; Assistant Professor of Radiology, Division of Body MRI, Department of Radiology, Mayo College of Medicine, Rochester, Minnesota

ALLEN T. BISHOP, MD, Professor of Orthopedic Surgery, Mayo Medical School; Chair, Division of Hand Surgery, Department of Orthopedic Surgery, Mayo Clinic, Rochester, Minnesota

ROBERT H. BROPHY, MD, Resident, Orthopedic Surgery, Hospital for Special Surgery, New York, New York

DAVID CHWEI-CHIN CHUANG, MD, Professor, Chairman, Department of Plastic Surgery, Chang Gung University Hospital, Taipei-Linkou, Taiwan

HENRI D. FOURNIER, MD, PhD, Doctor of Medicine, Service de Neurochirurgie, Centre Hospitalier Universitaire; Faculté de Médecine, Laboratoire d'Anatomie, Université d'Angers, Angers, France

C. MICHEL HARPER, MD, Professor of Neurology; Director of Electromyography Laboratory and Neuromuscular Clinic; Vice Chair, Department of Neurology, Mayo Clinic, Mayo Clinic College of Medicine, Rochester, Minnesota

DENISE KINLAW, PT, CHT, Assistant Professor of Physical Therapy, Mayo School of Health Sciences Program in Physical Therapy, Mayo Clinic, Rochester, Minnesota

DAVID G. KLINE, MD, Boyd Professor and Chairman, Department of Neurosurgery, Louisiana State University Health Sciences Center; MCLNO Hospital; Ochsner Hospital; and Touro Hospital, New Orleans, Louisiana

PHILIPPE MENEI, MD, PhD, Professor of Medicine, Service de Neurochirurgie, Centre Hospitalier Universitaire, Angers, France

PHILIPPE MERCIER, MD, Professor of Medicine, Service de Neurochirurgie, Centre Hospitalier Universitaire; Faculté de Médecine, Laboratoire d'Anatomie, Université d'Angers, Angers, France

STEVEN L. MORAN, MD, Assistant Professor, Division of Hand Surgery, Division of Plastic Surgery, and Department of Orthopedic Surgery, Mayo Clinic, Rochester, Minnesota

JOHN D. PORT, MD, PhD, Consultant and Assistant Professor of Radiology, Division of Neuroradiology, Department of Radiology, Mayo Clinic, Rochester, Minnesota

ALEXANDER Y. SHIN, MD, Associate Professor of Orthopedic Surgery, Orthopedic Hand and Microvascular Surgery, Mayo Medical School, Rochester, Minnesota

PANUPAN SONGCHAROEN, MD, Professor, Chief of Hand and Reconstructive Microsurgery Unit, Department of Orthopedic Surgery, Faculty of Medicine, Siriraj Hospital, Mahidol University, Bangkok, Thailand

ROBERT J. SPINNER, MD, Associate Professor, Departments of Neurologic Surgery, Orthopedics, and Anatomy, Mayo Clinic School of Medicine, Rochester, Minnesota

SCOTT P. STEINMANN, MD, Assistant Professor, Division of Hand Surgery, Department of Orthopedic Surgery, Mayo Clinic, Rochester, Minnesota

ROBERT L. TIEL, MD, Associate Professor, Department of Neurosurgery, Louisiana State University Health Sciences Center; MCLNO Hospital; Ochsner Hospital; and Touro Hospital, New Orleans, Louisiana

SCOTT W. WOLFE, MD, Attending Orthopedic Surgeon; Chief of Hand Service, Hospital for Special Surgery; Professor of Orthopedic Surgery, Cornell-Weill Medical Center, New York, New York

SAICHOL WONGTRAKUL, MD, Assistant Professor, Department of Orthopedic Surgery, Faculty of Medicine, Siriraj Hospital, Mahidol University, Bangkok, Thailand

CONTENTS

intraplexal neurotizations for preganglionic injuries (root avulsions) is discussed. A balanced perspective is presented, which considers the various surgical options, including promising, emerging techniques. New surgical strategies offer additional hope for patients with severe brachial plexus injuries to recover some useful function.

Functioning Free-Muscle Transfer for Brachial Plexus Injury

Allen T. Bishop

Functioning free-muscle transfers are now an important tool in management of patients with brachial plexus injuries. They are indicated for restoration of elbow flexion in patients with delayed presentation (those seen after 6–9 months). Double free-muscle transfers provide the possibility of grasp and release function of the hand with active elbow flexion and extension when combined with nerve transfers or grafts for restoration of shoulder motion, hand sensation, and triceps function.

Pre-/Postoperative Therapy for Adult Plexus Injury

Denise Kinlaw

The rehabilitation of patients who have sustained brachial plexus injuries is essential. Therapy is performed to maintain and increase range of motion, retard the rate of muscle atrophy, and re-educate the muscles once the reconstructive surgeries have been performed and reinnervation is verified. This article discusses pre- and postoperative therapy for these injuries.

Repair of Avulsed Ventral Nerve Roots by Direct Ventral Intraspinal Implantation after Brachial Plexus Injury

Henri D. Fournier, Philippe Mercier, and Philippe Menei

The avulsion of nerve roots associated with the brachial plexus results in lesions with a poor prognosis. These lesions involve the central nervous system and are therefore considered irreparable. The results of many experiments in animals have shown that if continuity can be re-established between the cervical cord and a denervated muscle or the distal end of its nerve, spinal motor neurons can regrow into a peripheral nerve graft, ultimately leading to the restoration of functional contraction. The current authors sought to prove that axons can regrow after intraspinal reimplantation of an avulsed nerve root, that such regrowth can lead to the recovery of function, and that the phenomenon should be focused on for the development of new surgical modalities to correct this serious condition. Partial reinnervation was obtained in the triceps, biceps, and deltoid muscles, and in the radial flexor muscle of the wrist, the exact pattern depending on the type of lesion and the type of graft. Treatment with neurotrophic factors represents a parallel line of research that might well help improve outcomes in spinal surgery to repair nerve root avulsion.

Index

FORTHCOMING ISSUES

RECENT ISSUES

HAND
CLINICS

Hand Clin 21 (2005) ix–x

Preface

Brachial Plexus Injuries in Adults

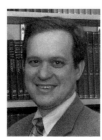
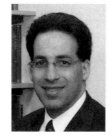
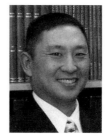

Allen T. Bishop, MD   Robert J. Spinner, MD   Alexander Y. Shin, MD
Guest Editors

The loss of upper extremity function following a traumatic brachial plexus injury causes devastating functional deficits that require complex surgical reconstruction. Because of advances and innovations in surgical techniques, it is now possible to reliably restore elbow flexion and shoulder stability, provided intervention is prompt. Recently, innovations have provided additional surgical reconstructive options that can be expected to improve functional outcomes. For example, methods are available that may, at times, restore basic grasp function in patients with lower plexus rupture or avulsion. Surgeons from all disciplines must be cognizant of these new possibilities and seek out additional training or partnerships across specialty boundaries to provide the best possible care in these devastating injuries. In many such reconstructive schemes, nerve transfer from multiple intra- and extraplexal donor nerves and microvascular transfer of functioning free muscles to the paralyzed limb are integral parts of the total reconstructive plan. The complexity and rigor of these procedures for both

the reconstructive team and patient are substantial. Successful outcomes require not only consideration of the nature of the plexus injury (including location, mechanism, and elapsed time from injury) and presence of associated injuries but also surgical expertise, practical operative-time constraints, and ability to provide and attend prolonged postoperative rehabilitation.

In this monograph, an international group of experts has distilled the current state-of-the-art in evaluation and management of brachial plexus injury. The concept for the monograph arose during a recent skills course held at the Mayo Clinic under the sponsorship of the American Society for Surgery of the Hand and endorsement of the Congress of Neurological Surgeons. The contributors are derived from that faculty and were selected based on their experience, knowledge, and innovative approach to the evaluation and management of this difficult problem.

It is our hope that these efforts will help clinicians caring for these unfortunate patients and, perhaps most important, to enable appropriate evaluation and timely referral to centers with expertise in brachial plexus care. Further, the experience of the authors should provide a means to allow surgeons to improve patient outcomes, and allow clinical investigators to further refine and improve the current state of the art.

Allen T. Bishop, MD
Division of Hand Surgery
Department of Orthopedic Surgery
Mayo Clinic
200 First Street, SW
Rochester, MN 55905, USA

E-mail address: bishop.allen@mayo.edu

Robert J. Spinner, MD
Departments of Neurologic Surgery,
Orthopedics, and Anatomy
Mayo Clinic School of Medicine
200 First Street, SW
Rochester, MN 55905, USA

E-mail address: spinner.robert@mayo.edu

Alexander Y. Shin, MD
Orthopedic Hand and Microvascular Surgery
Mayo Medical School
200 First Street, SW
Rochester, MN 55905, USA

E-mail address: shin.alexander@mayo.edu

ELSEVIER
SAUNDERS

Hand Clin 21 (2005) 1–11

HAND
CLINICS

Clinically Relevant Surgical Anatomy and Exposures of the Brachial Plexus

Alexander Y. Shin, MD[a],*, Robert J. Spinner, MD[b]

[a]Division of Hand Surgery, Department of Orthopedic Surgery, Mayo Clinic, Rochester, MN 55905, USA
[b]Department of Neurosurgery, Mayo Clinic, 200 First Street SW, Rochester, MN 55905, USA

Qu'ils n'oublient jamais que sans anatomie il n'y
a point de physiologie, point de chirurgie, point
de medicine.
 —J. Cruveilhier Traite d'Anatomie
Descriptive (1834)

The complex anatomy of the brachial plexus is
probably one of the most anxiety-provoking
subjects of medical school and residency curricula.
Surgical exploration of this area, however, de-
mands a clear and concise understanding of the
normal anatomy and its variations, including the
pathoanatomy. This article summarizes several
hundred years of literature on the anatomy of the
brachial plexus and then describes common surgical exposures to highlight the clinically relevant
features.

General overview of the brachial plexus

The brachial plexus runs within the interscalene
triangle (formed by the anterior scalene anteriorly,
the middle scalene posteriorly, and the superior
border of the first rib inferiorly). The brachial
plexus is also located within the posterior triangle
of the neck (formed by the sternocleidomastoid
(SCM) medially, the trapezius laterally, and the
clavicle inferiorly).

The brachial plexus is the network of nerves
that provides sensation and function to the upper
extremity. It is formed from the ventral primary
rami of the lowest four cervical nerve roots (C5–

C8) and that of the first thoracic nerve (T1;
Fig. 1). Although a frequent percentage of brachial plexuses have contributions from C4 (prefixed) [1–3] or T2 (postfixed) [2,4,5], these
contributions have little clinical significance.

The true form of the brachial plexus has been
best described by Kerr [2], who performed detailed anatomic dissections on 175 specimens (see
Fig. 1). In the "true form," the components of the
brachial plexus include the following: roots,
trunks, divisions, cords, and terminal branches.
Five roots form three trunks, which form six
divisions. These divisions form three cords, which
ultimately form five terminal branches. Roots and
trunks are found supraclavicularly; divisions are
located retroclavicularly; and cords and terminal
branches comprise the infraclavicular portion.

C5 and C6, and C8 and T1 roots merge to
form the upper and lower trunks. C7 becomes the
middle trunk. The point at which C5 and C6
merge is known as Erb's point. The upper trunk
trifurcates; the suprascapular nerve emerges from
the upper trunk and the two divisions are formed.
Each trunk divides into an anterior and posterior
division, and passes beneath the clavicle. The
posterior divisions from the trunks merge to
become the posterior cord, and the anterior
divisions of the upper and middle trunk merge
to form the lateral cord. The anterior division
from the lower trunk forms the medial cord. The
lateral cord splits into two terminal branches: the
musculocutaneous nerve and the lateral cord
contribution to the median nerve (the so-called
"sensory" part). The posterior cord forms the
axillary nerve and the radial nerve, and the medial
cord gives off the medial cord contribution to the

---

* Corresponding author.
 E-mail address: shin.alexander@mayo.edu
(A.Y. Shin).

0749-0712/05/$ - see front matter © 2005 Elsevier Inc. All rights reserved.
doi:10.1016/j.hcl.2004.09.006

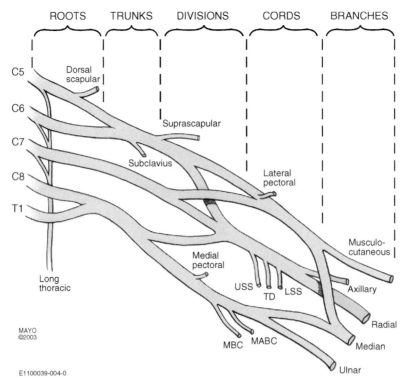

Fig. 1. The five portions of the brachial plexus are drawn out and separated into roots, trunks, division, cords, and terminal branches. LSS, lower subscapular nerve; MABC, medial antebrachial cutaneous nerve; MBC, medial brachial cutaneous nerve; TD, thoracodorsal nerve; USS, upper subscapular nerve. (Courtesy of the Mayo Foundation, Rochester, MN; with permission.)

median nerve (the so-called "motor" part) and the ulnar nerve.

There are a few terminal branches that come off the roots, trunks, and cords. The branches from the C5 root include the dorsal scapular nerve (rhomboid muscles), a branch to the phrenic nerve (with C3 and C4), and a branch to the long thoracic nerve (serratus anterior muscle). Branches from the C6 and C7 nerve also contribute to the long thoracic nerve. The branches off the upper trunk include the nerve to the subclavius muscle (clinically unimportant) and the suprascapular nerve. The lateral cord gives off the lateral pectoral nerve, whereas the posterior and medial cords each have three branches. The posterior cord typically gives off branches (proximal to distal) that include the upper subscapular nerve, the thoracodorsal nerve, and the lower subscapular nerve. The medial cord gives off the medial pectoral nerve, the medial brachial cutaneous nerve, and the medial antebrachial cutaneous nerve.

Common variations of the brachial plexus

Overall variations to the brachial plexus have been reported in more than 50% of cases [6]. The most common variations of the brachial plexus are related to the contributions of C4 and T2—the prefixed and postfixed brachial plexus. It has been estimated that C4 will be contributory in 28% to 62% of patients based on the dissection of brachial plexuses in cadavers (Fig. 2) [1–3]. The incidence of postfixed brachial plexuses ranges from 16% to 73% (Fig. 3) [2,4,5]. These branches range from very small to significant size.

Variations in the trunk level are relatively uncommon. Approximately 90% of upper trunks are formed by the confluence of C5 and C6, whereas in 8%, the upper trunk does not exist—C5 and C6 immediately split into divisions [2]. In the remaining 2% of upper trunks, C7 joined C5 and C6, and then divided into two parts. The middle trunk, which is the continuation of C7, was the normal finding in 93.7% of

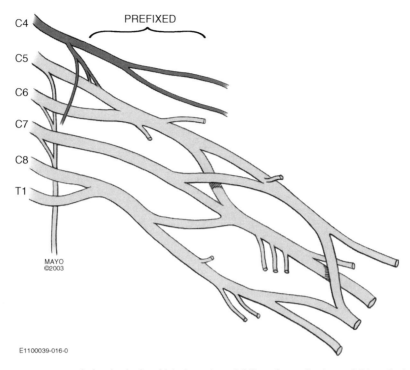

C4

PREFIXED

C5

C6

C7

C8

T1

MAYO
©2003

E1100039-016-0

Fig. 2. The most common variation in the brachial plexus is variability of contributions of C4 to the brachial plexus. This contribution of C4 nerve fibers to the brachial plexus is also known as a prefixed plexus. (Courtesy of the Mayo Foundation, Rochester, MN; with permission.)

specimens, whereas 3% of specimens had the middle trunk divide into two anterior divisions and one posterior division. The lower trunk was formed by the confluence of C8 and T1 in 95.4% of specimens [2].

A common variation of the lateral cord is for it to contribute to the ulnar nerve, and this variation has been reported to occur as frequently as 42.9% [2]. Another common variation is the size of the lateral cord contribution to the median nerve: when this is small, there is often a communication of the musculocutaneous nerve to the median nerve in the arm. The anatomy of the medial cord is relatively constant; it has been found to receive contributions from C8 and T1 in 94.6% of specimens and has few reported variations. The posterior cord has been reported to be absent in 20.8% of cadavers. In these specimens, the radial and axillary nerves arose independently from the brachial plexus.

Variations in the terminal branches are common. A discussion of every reported variation is beyond the scope of this article; only the most commonly encountered variations in the terminal branches are discussed. The suprascapular nerve

has been found to come from the upper trunk or its anterior or posterior divisions in more than 82% of specimens [2]. Occasionally, C4 may contribute directly to the suprascapular nerve. It also may be a terminal branch off of C5 with a small contribution to C6 [7]. The musculocutaneous nerve is commonly associated with variations. Kaplan and Spinner [8] noted that this nerve may seem absent because of a "double musculocutaneous nerve" or a combined median/musculocutaneous nerve. In 24% of specimens, there were C7 fibers present in the musculocutaneous nerve, and these fibers passed through a communication from the musculocutaneous nerve to the median nerve [8]. A low take-off of the musculocutaneous nerve from the lateral cord may confuse the surgeon, especially if he or she is using a small infraclavicular incision and does not identify this nerve branch within the surgical field. The posterior cord, with its terminal branches, the axillary and radial nerve, is also frequently variant. The radial nerve comes off the posterior cord in its classic position in 79% of specimens [2]. The variations include the radial nerve coming off the posterior division of the upper and middle trunk. The axillary nerve arises

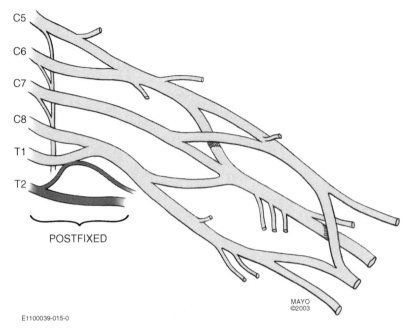

C5
C6
C7
C8
T1
T2

POSTFIXED

MAYO
©2003

E1100039-015-0

Fig. 3. The postfixed brachial plexus has a variable contribution of T2 to the brachial plexus. (Courtesy of the Mayo Foundation, Rochester, MN; with permission.)

in its classic position in 79.9% of specimens but can also arise from the upper and middle trunk divisions directly [2].

The axillary artery and its relationship to the brachial plexus elements may also be variant. Typically, at the level of the coracoid, the three cords are named for their anatomic relationship to the axillary artery: lateral, medial, and posterior cords (Fig. 4). Occasionally, a large superficial branch of the axillary artery will emerge between the medial and lateral cord contribution to the median nerve to course into the arm as a superficial radial, ulnar, brachial, or median artery. In addition to this variation, Miller [9] reported several vascular anomalous relationships (occurring in 8 of 480 specimens) where the median nerve below the convergence of the medial and lateral contributions was penetrated and divided by a branch of the axillary artery. Overall, the author reported 8% arterial and 4% venous variations associated with the brachial plexus.

Pathoanatomy

The anatomy of the rootlets, roots, and the vertebral foramen contributes to the type of injury (avulsion versus rupture) that is observed. At every level, each of the roots is formed by the joining of dorsal (sensory) rootlets and ventral (motor) rootlets off the spinal cord as they pass through the spinal foramen (Fig. 5A). The cell bodies of the sensory nerves lie within ganglia outside the spinal cord (ie, the dorsal root ganglia [DRG]). The rootlets that form the cervical roots are intraspinal and lack connective tissue or a meningeal envelope. This anatomic feature makes them vulnerable to traction and susceptible to avulsion at the level of the spinal cord. The meningeal layers are continuous as roots are formed. For example, the dura changes to epineurium within the foramen and is continuous with it. The extraspinal nerve within the foramen has a protective covering formed by the coalescence of the dura.

The spinal nerve is able to move freely within the foramina because it is not attached to it. The nerve roots run down chutes as they emerge from their respective foramina. There is a fibrous attachment of the spinal nerves to the transverse process that is seen in the fourth through seventh cervical root, which firmly attaches the nerves to the transverse process by an epineural sheath, prevertebral fascia, and fibrous slips. C8 and T1 do not have these connective tissue attachments. This anatomic arrangement explains the higher

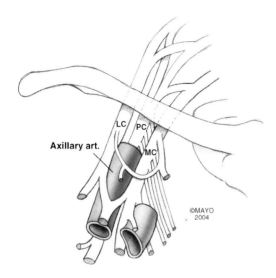

Fig. 4. The relationship of the axillary artery to the cords is an important anatomic relationship. The cords surround the axillary artery and are named for their position with respect to the axillary artery. LC, lateral cord; MC, medial cord; PC, posterior cord. (Courtesy of the Mayo Foundation, Rochester, MN; with permission.)

incidence of root avulsion in the lower two roots compared with the upper three roots.

When an injury causes the tearing of the rootlets from the spinal cord proximal to the DRG, the injury is classified as preganglionic or a root avulsion. Preganglionic injuries may occur centrally, where the nerve is torn directly from the spinal cord, or peripherally (an intradural rupture), where the injury is proximal to the DRG but remnants of the rootlets are still attached to the spinal cord (Fig. 5B). When an injury is distal to the DRG, it is called postganglionic. This type of stretch lesion may cause a disruption of the cervical root, or a rupture (Figs. 5C, D, and 6).

The implications that pre- versus postganglionic injuries have in surgical reconstruction are enormous. For practical purposes, the nerve connections in preganglionic injuries cannot be restored, and thus alternative nerves (eg, nerve transfers) must be used to reanimate the injured extremity. In postganglionic injuries, the nerve connections can be restored with interpositional nerve grafting to restore function.

Anatomic considerations of preganglionic injuries

Clinical examination and electrodiagnostic or imaging studies can provide evidence to support the anatomic considerations of a preganglionic injury. Physical examination may provide clues that the injury occurred at least close to the level of DRG (or foraminal level). These clues may include weakness of the rhomboids or the serratus anterior or the finding of a Horner's syndrome—the resultant loss of sympathetic outflow to the head and neck results, producing meiosis (small pupil), enophthalmos (sinking of the eyeball), ptosis (lid droop), and anhydrosis (dry eyes) of the ipsilateral face. The sympathetic ganglion for T1 lies in close proximity to the T1 root and provides sympathetic outflow to the head and neck. Because of this close association, avulsion of the T1 root typically causes interruption of the T1 sympathetic ganglion (Fig. 7). Fibrillations in paraspinal muscles (which are innervated by the dorsal primary rami, which arise at the exit of the intervertebral foramen) also would suggest a preganglionic injury. In addition, in preganglionic injury, sensory nerve conduction studies will often be preserved when, clinically, the patient is insensate, because the sensory nerve cell body is intact within the DRG. Chest radiographs may show an elevated hemidiaphragm (from phrenic nerve dysfunction) or cervical films may show transverse process fractures. A CT-myelogram may show pseudomeningoceles or an MRI may reveal absent nerve rootlets.

Anatomic considerations of postganglionic injuries

The anatomic configuration of the brachial plexus predisposes it to injury at sites where it is relatively fixed to the surrounding tissues. These points can occur when branches take off from larger nerve structures, or when nerves are tethered by soft tissue (eg, muscles, ligaments, tendons) or osseous structures. One of the more well know points of tethering is that of Erb's point, where the suprascapular nerve comes off the upper trunk. Because the upper trunk is relatively tethered, and the suprascapular nerve and the division of the upper trunk are relatively free, it is a common site of a rupture. The suprascapular nerve is also bound at the suprascapular notch, and with displacement of the scapula from trauma, the suprascapular nerve can sustain a rupture at this location as well. The clavicle can also contribute to brachial plexus injuries at the level of the divisions. The axillary nerve, as it passes posteriorly after its take-off from the posterior cord, is tethered by the soft tissue, which is often a site for its rupture. In addition, the axillary nerve can be injured within the quadrangular space.

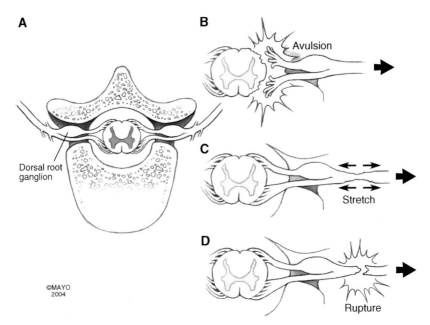

Fig. 5. (*A*) The root is made from contributions from dorsal (sensory) rootlets and ventral (motor) rootlets that emerge from the spinal cord and coalesce into the cervical root and emerges from the vertebral foramen. It is important to understand that the cell bodies of the dorsal (sensory) portion lie within the DRG. When an injury occurs and the rootlets are torn out of the spinal cord, the injury is classified as preganglionic, because it occurs proximal to the DRG. (*B*) This type of injury is also known as an avulsion. (*C, D*) When the cervical root is injured or becomes discontinuous distal to the DRG, the injury is classified as a postganglionic injury. (Courtesy of the Mayo Foundation, Rochester, MN; with permission.)

Operative approaches to the brachial plexus

Supraclavicular brachial plexus

The patient is placed supine, occasionally placed in a modified beach chair position to facilitate a posterior approach to the shoulder or arm. A folded sheet is placed beneath the scapula. The neck is extended gently and turned to the opposite side. A bump is also placed beneath the buttock to externally rotate one leg (should a sural nerve graft be desirable). The neck, shoulder, entire limb, chest, and both legs are prepared and draped.

The supraclavicular brachial plexus can be approached through an incision paralleling the lateral border of the SCM. This approach may be combined with an incision along the clavicle by itself and one inferiorly in the deltopectoral groove for exposure of the infraclavicular brachial plexus. For cosmetic reasons, the current authors prefer displaying the supraclavicular brachial plexus through a transverse incision placed in a skin crease several fingers above the clavicle (Fig. 8). The platysma is divided, and generous

subplatysmal flaps are raised, which enhance the exposure. The external jugular vein is retracted. The border of the SCM muscle is identified and its clavicular head is either retracted medially or released (and later repaired). The supraclavicular fat pad is dissected and mobilized laterally. The omohyoid muscle is either retracted, or tagged and divided for later reapproximation. Nerves of the cervical plexus may be seen during the superficial exposure, and they can be traced to C3 and C4 origins. These branches should be preserved if at all possible to prevent the potential formation of painful neuroma, if transected. If the carotid artery or internal jugular vein is identified, then the dissection is too medial.

The phrenic nerve should be identified on the surface of the anterior scalene muscle and carefully mobilized proximally. The phrenic nerve runs inferiorly and medially (the only major nerve to take this course). This nerve is usually functional, and it can be stimulated intraoperatively. The phrenic nerve is traced proximally, and at the lateral edge of the anterior scalene, its C5 contribution is identified. Once C5 is identified and

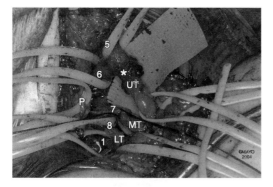

Fig. 6. Left supraclavicular exposure in this patient with an obstetric brachial plexus palsy revealed a neuroma-in-continuity (*) of the upper trunk (UT) and a rupture of the middle trunk (MT). (Both ends were tagged with sutures.) The C8, T1, and lower trunk (LT) were scarred but conducted nerve action potentials. P, phrenic nerve. (Courtesy of the Mayo Foundation, Rochester, MN; with permission.)

mobilized, C6 is identified caudal and dorsal to C5 (Fig. 9A). The C5 and C6 root then join to form the upper trunk. The upper trunk can be followed distally to expose the suprascapular nerve and the anterior and posterior divisions. The clavicle can be mobilized if retroclavicular exposure is necessary, and retracted downward. The suprascapular artery and vein should be ligated and the subclavius muscle divided.

For proximal exposure of the roots, the anterior scalene muscle is divided. This step allows

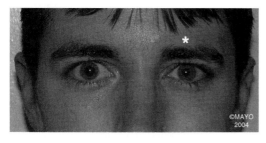

Fig. 7. Because of the close anatomic relationship between the T1 root and the T1 sympathetic ganglion, avulsions of the T1 root often result in injury to the T1 sympathetic ganglion, which has outflow to the head and neck. The disruption of the T1 sympathetic outflow results in Horner's syndrome: meiosis (small pupil), enophthalmos (sinking of the eyeball), ptosis (lid droop), and anhydrosis (dry eyes) of the ipsilateral face. In the clinical example shown, the asterisk identifies the injured side. (Courtesy of the Mayo Foundation, Rochester, MN; with permission.)

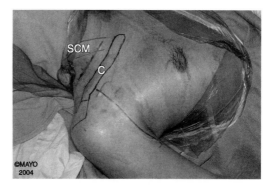

Fig. 8. Planned incisions for right supraclavicular and infraclavicular exposures. C, clavicle. (Courtesy of the Mayo Foundation, Rochester, MN; with permission.)

exposure at a foraminal level. Leksell rongeurs can assist in biting away the tip of the transverse processes for more proximal exposure, if this is deemed necessary. Care must be taken to avoid injury to the vertebral artery within the foramen transversarium. Venous bleeding must also be controlled. Proximal branches to the dorsal scapular nerve (C5 ± C4) and the long thoracic (C5–C7) may be seen. Dissection on the undersurface of C6 may expose the long thoracic nerve before it passes through the middle scalene.

The middle trunk and C7 are found more medially and deeper to the upper trunk (Fig. 9B). The transverse cervical artery may need to be ligated. When exposing the lower trunk, C8 and T1, the subclavian artery (posterior to the scalene anterior) and subclavian vein (anterior to the scalene anterior) should be identified and mobilized (Fig. 9C, D). These neural elements embrace the first rib, so special care should be maintained during their proximal exposure to avoid injury to the pleura. The take-off of the vertebral artery should be kept in mind with dissection of the lower neural elements. The thoracic duct may be vulnerable, especially on left-sided exposures.

The spinal accessory nerve may be identified 1 cm above the point where the great auricular nerve wraps around the SCM (near the area where iatrogenic injury to it may occur during posterior triangle lymph node biopsies). The authors typically do not identify it as part of their supraclavicular brachial plexus exposure. When they use the spinal accessory nerve as a nerve transfer, however, they prefer to identify it more distally, along the medial border of the trapezius muscle, above the clavicle. Here, the authors find that the nerve is easier to locate and closer to where they wish to transect it, deep at the inferior portion

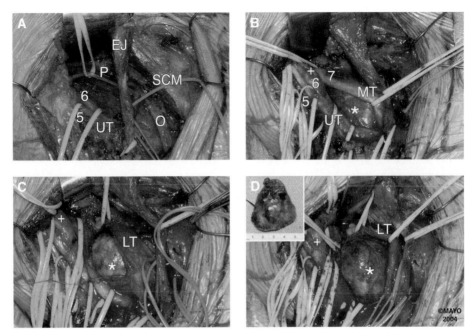

Fig. 9. Right supraclavicular exposure in an adult with schwannomatosis. The patient presented with ulnar-sided hand pain and a large neck mass, although neurologic examination was normal. MRI showed a large nerve sheath tumor involving the lower trunk (LT) and a smaller one arising from C6. (*A*) Initial dissection shows that the phrenic nerve (P) has been mobilized. It was used to identify C5, C6 and the upper trunk (UT). (*B*) C7 and the middle trunk (MT), which were displaced by the large tumor (*) have been mobilized. The smaller tumor can be seen within C6 (*plus sign*). (*C*) After proximal and distal control of neural elements has been obtained, the tumor (*) involving the LT is exposed. (*D*) The large tumor (*) is resected and the LT is preserved. The smaller lesion (*plus sign*) was then resected at a fascicular level from C6. Full neurologic function was maintained. Pathology confirmed two schwannomas (inset shows the larger resected mass). +, smaller tumor lesion; *, larger tumor lesion; EJ, external jugular vein; O, omohyoid. (Courtesy of the Mayo Foundation, Rochester, MN; with permission.)

of the trapezius. A long segment of nerve can be harvested (ie, long enough to extend several centimeters below the clavicle). Still, proximal branches to the upper and midtrapezius are preserved.

Retroclavicular brachial plexus

Exposure to the retroclavicular brachial plexus can be facilitated by mobilization of the clavicle and by proximal and distal exposure of the brachial plexus. In select cases in which generous exposure of the divisions is necessary, the authors use a clavicular osteotomy. They contour a low-contour reconstruction plate and predrill it before osteotomizing the clavicle, because this technique improves union rates.

Infraclavicular brachial plexus

An incision is made from the clavicle down using the deltopectoral interval (deltoid and pectoralis major). A portion of the clavicular

attachment of the pectoralis major and deltoid may be released to facilitate exposure. The intermuscular interval is most easily identified proximally, which may be useful in revision surgery. The cephalic vein is mobilized. The authors prefer to retract it laterally. Distal exposure of the infraclavicular brachial plexus is enhanced by releasing the uppermost portion of the pectoralis major insertion. The authors typically do not release the pectoralis major insertion, but if this is necessary for broad exposure, they recommend leaving a small cuff of tendon behind and tagging it for later repair.

The deltopectoral interval is deepened. The pectoralis minor is identified arising from the coracoid and inserting on the ribs. It is tagged and divided through its tendon, although in some cases it may be retracted. The infraclavicular brachial plexus is visualized just beneath the fat pad. The lateral cord is identified first. It can be traced to the musculocutaneous nerve (although this branch may arise more distally and, on some occasions, not be seen in a standard infraclavicular approach) and the lateral cord contribution to the median nerve. The axillary artery should be mobilized and protected. Small branches may need to be ligated. The thoracoacromial trunk can be used for the arterial repair of a free-muscle transfer. The axillary vein lies more medially. The posterior cord and its terminal branches can be identified more deeply after the lateral cord, musculocutaneous nerve, and branch to the coracobrachialis muscles have been neurolysed and the artery sufficiently mobilized. The release of the coracobrachialis tendon may improve exposure of the axillary nerve. The medial cord can be identified medial to the axillary artery. The terminal branches of the medial cord can then be identified easily. The "M" (formed by the terminal branches of the lateral and medial cords) is then entirely visualized. The median nerve is formed just below the level of the coracoid.

The infraclavicular brachial plexus dissection is usually fairly easy under routine situations where the injury has occurred in the supraclavicular region. When the infraclavicular brachial plexus is scarred either from injury or previous surgery (eg, vascular repair), however, dissection may be difficult.

Medial exposure of nerve branches in proximal arm

Several terminal branches can be identified quickly by a separate short longitudinal incision in the proximal medial arm. This step may be useful, especially when performing nerve transfers (eg, the Oberlin transfer) [10,11]. Alternatively, extension of the deltopectoral incision into the proximal arm may be performed. The medial antebrachial cutaneous nerve, median nerve (the largest neural structure in this exposure is found deep to the brachial artery), and ulnar nerve can be identified within several centimeters of each other. The musculocutaneous nerve can be found between the biceps and coracobrachialis muscles. Its branches to the biceps, brachialis, and lateral antebrachial cutaneous nerve can then be isolated [12].

Posterior approaches

Posterior subscapular approach

The posterior subscapular approach, popularized by Dr. David Kline, is especially useful when very proximal exposure is needed, especially for C7

through T1 [13,14]. It may be particularly helpful for select cases, such as revision cases (eg, after supraclavicular approach for thoracic outlet surgery) or tumors involving lower plexal elements.

The patient is placed prone with rolls beneath the chest and transversely under the shoulders. The patient is placed in a reverse Trendelenberg position. The arm on the affected side must be permitted to move freely so as not to limit scapular mobilization. A lazy-S–shaped parascapular incision is made between the medial edge of the scapula and the thoracic spinous processes and is extended to the midneck region. The trapezius is divided. The rhomboids and, at times, the levator scapulae, are divided and tagged, and the serratus posterior is sectioned. A thoracotomy retractor is placed between the scapula and paraspinous muscles. The ribs are exposed. The scalenes are detached from the first rib insertion. The first rib is removed near the costovertebral junction. The neural elements and subclavian vessels are identified. Care must be taken to avoid injury to the spinal accessory, long thoracic, and dorsal scapular nerves (the phrenic nerve lies anteriorly). Very proximal exposure can be obtained by performing foraminotomies and even partial laminectomies, as appropriate. This approach also allows good exposure to divisions.

Meticulous attention must be placed to anatomic closure. The surgeon must check for potential pneumothorax and treat appropriately with a chest tube. Tagging sutures (Vicryl-0) should reapproximate muscular layers anatomically.

Posterior approach to the suprascapular nerve

The suprascapular nerve can be exposed posteriorly when the site of the lesion is at the suprascapular notch region. This exposure can be obtained when the patient is in a semilateral position, when performed as part of an anterior brachial plexus (or suprascapular nerve) exposure, or prone, when it is used for an entrapment lesion. A 6- to 8-cm incision is made 1 cm superior to the scapular spine. The posterior incision is made centered at the level of the coracoid process, which can be palpated anteriorly. The trapezius muscle may be split in line with its fibers or it may be taken down from the scapular spine. A fat pad is seen. The atrophied supraspinatus muscle is reflected inferiorly. The suprascapular nerve passes obliquely through the transverse scapular ligament. The ligament is released. The operative

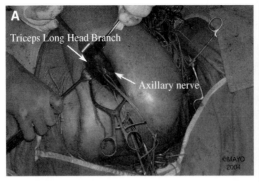
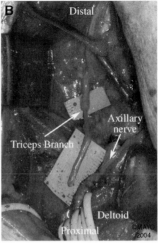

Fig. 10. (*A*) Posterior approach for a triceps branch to axillary nerve transfer, with the triceps branch to the long head identified and the axillary nerve identified. (*B*). A close-up view shows the triceps branch to the long head already divided distally and flipped proximally. (Courtesy of the Mayo Foundation, Rochester, MN; with permission.)

microscope may be helpful, as much for the lighting as the magnification.

Posterior approach to the axillary and radial nerves

Posterior exposure of the axillary and radial nerves may be helpful when adequate distal exposure of these nerves cannot be obtained anteriorly. The authors also have found this exposure especially useful when performing a nerve transfer suturing a triceps branch to the axillary nerve. When this approach is being considered, they place a bump under the patient so that they may obtain a more lateral approach.

A longitudinal incision is made along the posterior surface of the proximal arm that extends to the lateral edge of the scapula. The deltoid is retracted anteriorly. The interval between the long and lateral heads of the triceps is developed. The superior lateral brachial cutaneous nerve can be helpful if seen in the superficial dissection and if traced deep to the main axillary nerve. The axillary nerve and its branches (and the posterior humeral circumflex artery) can be identified as the nerve emerges from the quadrangular space, superior to the teres major. The radial nerve and its branches (and the profunda brachii artery) can be seen inferior to the teres major [15,16] (Fig. 10).

Summary

A clear understanding of the anatomy of the brachial plexus and its relationship to vascular,

skeletal and muscular anatomy is essential for any surgery of this area. Adequate exposure and delineation of the pathology will allow for accurate treatment of the brachial plexus lesion(s).

References

[1] Jachimowicz J. Les variation du plexus brachial [resume]. E. Loth, translator. Mem Anat A Univ Varsoviensis 1925;246–82.

[2] Kerr A. Brachial plexus of nerves in man. The variations in its formation and branches. Am J Anat 1918; 23:285.

[3] Senecail B. Le plexus brachial de l'Homme. In: These Reims, vol. 66. 1975.

[4] Adolphi H. Uber das Verhalten der zweiten Brustnerven zum plexus brachialis beim Menschen. Anat Anz 1898;15:25–36.

[5] Hirasawa K. Uber den Pelxus Brachialis Mitterlung die Wurzeln des Plexus Brachial. In: Impressio separata ex actis Scholac Medicinalis. Paris: Univeritatis Imperialis Kiotoensis; 1927.

[6] Uysal II, Seker M, Karabulut AK, et al. Brachial plexus variations in human fetuses. Neurosurgery 2003;53:676.

[7] Hovelacque A. Anatomie des nerfs craniens et rachidiens et du systeme grand sympathique. Paris: Doins.

[8] Kaplan E, Spinner M. Normal and anomalous innervation patterns in the upper extremity. In: Omer G, Spinner M, editors. Management of peripheral nerve problems. Philadelphia: WB Saunders; 1980. p. 75–99.

[9] Miller R. Observations upon the arrangement of the axillary and brachial plexus. Am J Anat 1939;64:143.

[10] Loy S, Bhatia A, Asfazadourian H, et al. Ulnar nerve fascicle transfer onto to the biceps muscle nerve in C5-C6 or C5-C6-C7 avulsions of the brachial plexus. Eighteen cases [in French]. Ann Chir Main Memb Super 1997;16:275.

[11] Oberlin C, Beal D, Leechavengvongs S, et al. Nerve transfer to biceps muscle using a part of ulnar nerve for C5-C6 avulsion of the brachial plexus: anatomical study and report of four cases. J Hand Surg [Am] 1994;19:232.

[12] Chiarapattanakom P, Leechavengvongs S, Witoonchart K, et al. Anatomy and internal topography of the musculocutaneous nerve: the nerves to the biceps and brachialis muscle. J Hand Surg [Am] 1998;23:250.

[13] Dubuisson AS, Kline DG, Weinshel SS. Posterior subscapular approach to the brachial plexus. Report of 102 patients. J Neurosurg 1993;79:319.

[14] Kline DG, Kott J, Barnes G, et al. Exploration of selected brachial plexus lesions by the posterior subscapular approach. J Neurosurg 1978; 49:872.

[15] Leechavengvongs S, Witoonchart K, Uerpairojkit C, et al. Nerve transfer to deltoid muscle using the nerve to the long head of the triceps, part II: a report of 7 cases. J Hand Surg [Am] 2003;28:633.

[16] Witoonchart K, Leechavengvongs S, Uerpairojkit C, et al. Nerve transfer to deltoid muscle using the nerve to the long head of the triceps, part I: an anatomic feasibility study. J Hand Surg [Am] 2003;28:628.

ELSEVIER
SAUNDERS

Hand Clin 21 (2005) 13–24

HAND
CLINICS

Adult Brachial Plexus Injuries: Mechanism, Patterns of Injury, and Physical Diagnosis

Steven L. Moran, MD[a],*, Scott P. Steinmann, MD[b], Alexander Y. Shin, MD[b]

[a]*Division of Hand Surgery, Division of Plastic Surgery, Department of Orthopedic Surgery, Mayo Clinic, 200 First Street, Rochester, MN 55905, USA*
[b]*Division of Hand Surgery, Department of Orthopedic Surgery, Mayo Clinic, 200 First Street, Rochester, MN 55905, USA*

Brachial plexus lesions frequently lead to significant physical disability, psychologic distress, and socioeconomic hardship. Adult brachial plexus injuries can be caused by various mechanisms, including penetrating injuries, falls, and motor vehicle trauma. Often the diagnosis is delayed or ignored as the practitioner waits for some recovery. Expedient diagnosis and testing is the best means of maximizing functional return. Evaluators must remember that muscles will begin to undergo atrophy and lose motor end plates as soon as the proximal injury occurs. Thus, early surgical intervention is the best predictor of a successful outcome.

Incidence and cause

The number of brachial plexus injuries that occur each year is difficult to ascertain; however, with the advent of more extreme sporting activities and more powerful motor sports, and the increasing number of survivors of high-speed motor vehicle accidents, the number of plexus injuries continues to rise in many centers throughout the world [1–6]. Most patients with brachial plexus injuries are men and boys aged between 15 and 25 years [5,7–9]. Based on his nearly two decades of work with more than 1000 patients with brachial plexus injuries, Narakas [10] stated that 70% of traumatic brachial plexus injuries

occur secondary to motor vehicle accidents and, of these, 70% involve motorcycles or bicycles. In addition, 70% of cycle riders will have other major injuries.

Classification of nerve injury

To understand the requirements for surgery, it is first necessary to review the patterns of nerve injury. Historically, nerve injuries have been described using the Seddon and Sunderland classification scheme. Seddon's [11] original classification scheme described three possibilities for a dysfunctional nerve: neuropraxia, axonotmesis, or neurotmesis. A neuropraxia is present when there is a conduction block at the site of injury, but no macroscopic injury to the nerve. There may be a demyelinating injury, but Wallerian degeneration does not take place distal to the zone of injury. As soon as the block is resolved, nerve function to the target organ will normalize. The recovery time may extend from hours to months, depending on the extent and severity of the injury to the myelin covering. Physical examination will not show a Tinel's sign. Electrodiagnostic studies will show no conduction across the area of injury but will show normal conduction distal to the area of injury; this finding is unique to neuropraxias [12]. In axonotmesis, the axon or nerve fibers are ruptured, but the epineurium and perineurium remain intact. Wallerian degeneration will occur distal to the injury, but regeneration in the surviving proximal stump is still possible and should occur at a rate of 1 to 4 mm per day

* Corresponding author.
E-mail address: moran.steven@mayo.edu (S.L. Moran).

[13]. In neurotmesis, the entire nerve trunk is ruptured and axonal continuity cannot be restored. Without surgical intervention, this injury pattern will heal as a nonfunctional neuroma.

Sunderland expanded Seddon's classification scheme into five categories after observing that some patients with axonotmeses recovered, whereas others did not [12]. These new categories were added to better describe the condition of the endoneurium; if the endoneurium remains intact, the nerve has the potential to regenerate to its target organ.

Sunderland's first-degree injuries are the same as Seddon's neuropraxia. A second-degree injury involves a rupture of the axon, but the basal lamina or endoneurium remains intact, which allows for the possibility of recovery following Wallerian degeneration. A Tinel's sign will be noted on examination. The examiner should begin percussion distal to the injury site and note the most distal extent of the Tinel's sign. This distal Tinel's sign marks the site of the regenerating nerve cone. The site of the original trauma may show percussive sensitivity for several months, which should not be mistaken for advancing nerve fibers or a nonfunctional neuroma without first testing distally. Recovery from second-degree injuries should be complete unless the injury is so proximal to the target organ that muscle atrophy or motor end-plate degeneration occurs within the period of nerve regrowth. Third-degree lesions involve injury to the endoneurium with preservation of the perineurium. With disruption of the endoneurium, scarring will occur and full recovery is unlikely. Fourth-degree injury involves rupture of the fasciculi with disruption of the perineurium. The nerve is in continuity but scarring will likely prevent regeneration. A Tinel's sign will be present at the site of injury but will not advance. A fifth-degree injury is defined as complete transection of the nerve and epineurium. Findings are similar to a fourth-degree injury. There will be no advancement of the Tinel's sign and there will be no evidence of reinnervation with electrodiagnostic testing.

Mackinnon [12] has popularized an additional "sixth-degree" injury pattern, which represents a mixed pattern of nerve injury encompassing all degrees of injury: neuropraxia, axonotmesis, and neurotmesis. Some fascicles within the zone of injury may recover, whereas others will not. This finding complicates the diagnosis. This injury pattern is often seen in cases of traction. Traction forces on the nerve initially lengthen the epineurium and perineurium. The fasciculi are then stretched, reducing the nerves' cross-sectional area, which raises intrafascicular pressure. Before axonal rupture, the epineurium and perineurium rupture and strip off the nerve. Axons tend to rupture over several centimeters, with the larger fascicles breaking first [13]. Long areas of fibrosis and scarring are produced, which inhibit nerve regeneration. The successful repair of these types of injuries often involves intraoperative nerve stimulation to identify which portions of the nerve are capable of spontaneous recovery and those portions of the nerve which require resection, grafting, or neurotization. In these cases, definitive surgery is often delayed up to 3 months until the physician can determine the potential for nerve recovery.

Mechanism and pathoanatomy

Most adult brachial plexus pathology is caused by closed trauma. Nerve injury in these cases is from traction and compression, with traction accounting for 95% of injuries [14]. Following a traction injury, the nerves may rupture, be avulsed at the level of the spinal cord, or be significantly stretched but remain intact (Fig. 1). Following are five possible levels where the nerve can be injured (Fig. 2):

1. The root
2. The anterior branches of the spinal nerves
3. The trunk
4. The cord
5. The peripheral nerve

Root injuries may be further localized with respect to the dorsal root ganglion (DRG). Postganglionic (infraganglionic) injuries are located distal to the DRG, whereas preganglionic (supraganglionic) lesions are located proximal to the DRG. With both types of lesions, patients present with loss of muscle function. In preganglionic injuries, the nerve has been avulsed from the spinal cord separating the motor nerve fibers from the motor cell bodies in the anterior horn cells. The sensory fibers and cell bodies are still connected at the DRG; however, the efferent fibers entering the dorsal spinal column have been disrupted. Thus, sensory nerve action potentials (SNAPs) are preserved in patients with supraganglionic injuries. In postganglionic injuries, both the motor and sensory nerve cells have been disrupted so there will be abnormalities in both motor action potentials and SNAPs (see Fig. 1) [15]. At present, the repair of preganglionic

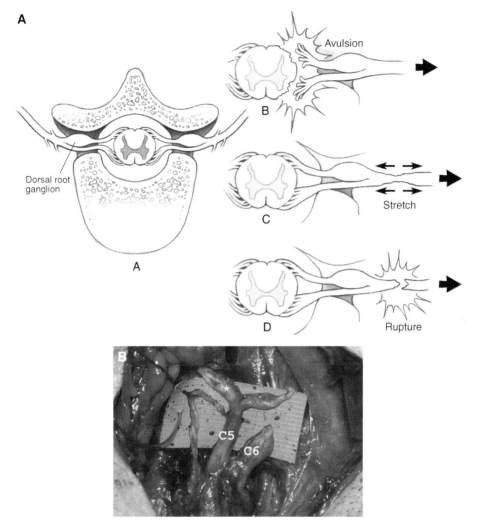

Fig. 1. (*A*) Anatomy of the brachial plexus roots and types of injury. Image A shows the roots are formed by the coalescence of the ventral (motor) and dorsal (sensory) rootlets as they pass through the spinal foramen. The DRG holds the cell bodies of the sensory nerves, whereas the cell bodies for the ventral nerves lie within the spinal cord. There are three types of injury that can occur: avulsion injuries, as shown in image B, pull the rootlets out of the spinal cord; stretch injuries, as shown in image C, attenuate the nerve; and ruptures, as shown in D, result in a complete discontinuity of the nerve. When the injury to the nerve is proximal to the DRG, it is called preganglionic, and when it is distal to the DRG, it is called postganglionic. (*B*) A clinical example of a preganglionic injury (root avulsion) and a postganglionic injury. In this patient, the C5 root is avulsed with its dorsal and ventral rootlets. The asterisk shows the DRG. The C6 root is inferior and demonstrates a rupture at the root level. (Courtesy of the Mayo Foundation, Rochester, MN; with permission.)

injuries requires a neurotization procedure. Post-ganglionic injuries may be amenable to surgical repair or grafting.

Root avulsions

Root avulsions are present in 75% of cases of supraclavicular lesions; multiple root avulsions have become more frequent over the past 25 years. There are two mechanisms for avulsion injuries: peripheral and central. Peripheral avulsion injuries are more common, whereas central avulsion injuries are rare and usually the result of direct cervical trauma (Figs. 3 and 4).

The peripheral mechanism occurs when traction forces on the arm overcome the fibrous

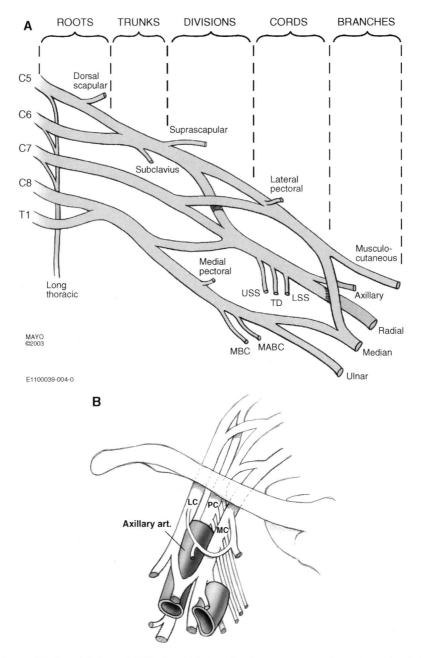

Fig. 2. Anatomy of the brachial plexus. (*A*) The brachial plexus has five major segments: roots, trunks, divisions, cords, and branches. The clavicle overlies the divisions. The roots and trunks are considered the supraclavicular plexus, whereas the cords and branches are considered the infraclavicular plexus. (*B*) The relationship between the axillary artery and the cords is shown. The cords are named for their anatomic relationship to the axillary artery: medial, lateral, and posterior. LC, lateral cord; LSS, lower sub scapular nerve; MABC, medial antibrachial cutaneous nerve; MBC, medial brachial cutaneous nerve; MC, medial cord; PC, posterior cord; TD, thoracodorsal; USS, upper sub scapular nerve. (Courtesy of the Mayo Foundation, Rochester, MN; with permission.)

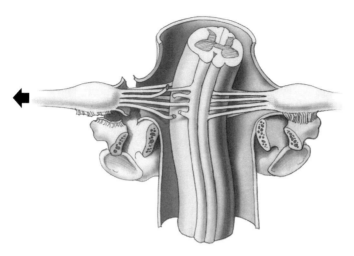

Fig. 3. Peripheral mechanism of avulsion. Peripheral avulsions occur when there is a traction force to the arm and the fibrous supports around the rootlets are avulsed. The epidural sleeve may be pulled out of the spinal canal, creating a pseudomeningocele.

supports around the rootlets. Anterior roots may be avulsed with or without the posterior rootlets. The epidural sac may tear without complete avulsion of the rootlets. Different injury types account for the different patterns seen on myelography. The epidural cone moves into the foraminal canal with peripheral avulsions (Fig. 5). Nagano et al [16,17] have classified avulsion and partial avulsion patterns based on findings at the time of myelogram. The nerve roots of C5 and C6 have strong fascial attachments at the spine and are less commonly avulsed in comparison to the nerve roots of C7 through T1.

The central mechanism of root avulsion is the result of the spinal cord moving longitudinally or transversely following significant cervical trauma. Spinal bending within the medullary canal induces avulsion of the rootlets [18]. The root remains fixed in the foramen and the epidural sleeve is not ruptured (see Fig. 4).

Injury patterns

Any combination of avulsion, rupture, or stretch may occur following a brachial plexus injury; however, certain patterns are more

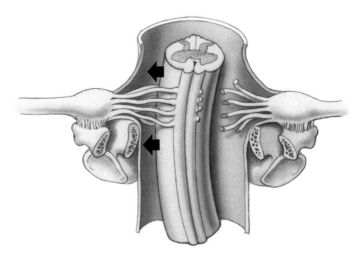

Fig. 4. Central mechanism of avulsion. Central avulsions occur from direst cervical trauma. The spinal cord is moved transversely or longitudinally, causing a sheering and spinal bending that results in an avulsion of nerve rootlets.

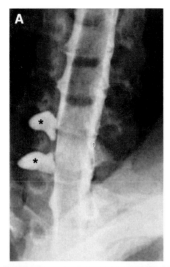

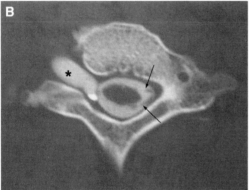

Fig. 5. Myelography and CT myelography can be instrumental in determining the level of nerve injury. If a pseudomeningocele (*) is present, there is a greater likelihood of a nerve root avulsion. (*A*) Multiple root avulsions (*) are clearly seen by CT myelogram. (*B*). The arrows on the opposite side of the avulsion (*) show the normal dorsal and ventral rootlet outline of the uninjured side. Notice how these outlines are missing on the injured side. (Courtesy of the Mayo Foundation, Rochester, MN; with permission.)

prevalent. Brachial plexus lesions most frequently affect the supraclavicular region rather than the retroclavicular or infraclavicular levels. The roots and trunks are more commonly injured in comparison to the divisions, cords, or terminal branches. Double-level injuries can occur and should be included in the differential. In the supraclavicular region, traction injuries occur when the head and neck are violently moved away from the ipsilateral shoulder, often resulting in an injury to the C5, C6 roots or upper trunk (Fig. 6). Traction to the brachial plexus can also

occur with violent arm motion. When the arm is abducted over the head with significant force, traction will occur within the lower elements of the brachial plexus (C8–T1 roots or lower trunk; Fig. 7).

Distal infraclavicular lesions are usually caused by violent injury to the shoulder girdle. These lesions can be associated with axillary arterial rupture. Biomechanically for a cord to rupture, it must be firmly fixed at both ends. The two major mechanisms for rupture are the anterior medial dislocation of the glenohumeral joint and traction of the upper arm with forced abduction [13]. The nerves become injured between two points at which the nerve is either fixed, restrained by surrounding structures, or where it changes direction. Suprascapular, axillary, and musculocutaneous nerves are susceptible to rupture because they are tethered within the glenohumeral area at the scapular notch and coracobrachialis. Physicians must always consider the possibility of a double crush at the scapular notch and the musculocutaneous nerve at the coracobrachialis. Rupture of the ulnar nerve at the level of the humerus or elbow and median nerve rupture at the level of the elbow are also possible.

Approximately 70% to 75% of injuries are found in the supraclavicular region. Approximately 75% of these injuries involve an injury to the entire plexus (C5–T1); in addition, 20% to 25% of injuries involve damage to the nerve roots of C5 through C7 and 2% to 35% of injuries have isolated supraclavicular injury patterns to C8 and T1. Panplexal injuries usually involve a C5-C6 rupture with a C7-T1 root avulsion. The remaining 25% of plexus injuries are infraclavicular.

Other mechanisms

Though less common than closed injuries, open injuries do occur. If the mechanism results in sharp division (eg, by means of a knife), direct repair may be possible. Iatrogenic injuries have been reported from multiple surgical procedures, including mastectomy, first rib resection, and subclavian carotid bypass [19–21]. Emergency exploration for open trauma is usually only warranted in cases of vascular injury or sharp laceration. Lower truck injuries are more likely to have concomitant vascular injuries. Open injuries caused by gunshot wounds are best managed conservatively because the nerve in these injuries is rarely transected [9].

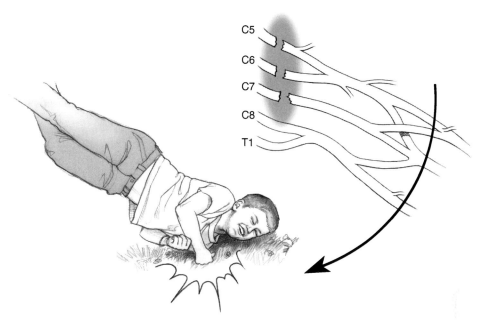

Fig. 6. Upper brachial plexus injuries occur when the head and neck are violently moved away from the ipsilateral shoulder. The shoulder is forced downward whereas the head is forced to the opposite side. The result is a stretch, avulsion, or rupture of the upper roots (C5, C6, C7), with preservation of the lower roots (C8, T1). (Courtesy of the Mayo Foundation, Rochester, MN; with permission.)

Physical examination

A patient with a brachial plexus injury is often seen in conjunction with significant trauma. This additional trauma can potentially delay diagnosis of any existing nerve injury until the patient is stabilized and resuscitated. A high index of suspicion for a brachial plexus injury should be maintained when examining a patient in the emergency department who has a significant shoulder girdle injury, first rib injuries, or axillary arterial injuries. Often, the patient is obtunded or sedated in the emergency setting and careful observation therefore is necessary as the patient becomes more coherent.

A detailed examination of the brachial plexus and its terminal branches can be performed in a few minutes on an awake and cooperative patient. The median, ulnar, and radial nerves can be evaluated by examining finger and wrist motion. Further up the arm, elbow flexion and extension can be examined to determine musculocutaneous and high radial nerve function. An examination of shoulder abduction can determine the function of the axillary nerve, a branch of the posterior cord. An injury to the posterior cord may affect deltoid function and the muscles innervated by the radial nerve. Thus, examination of wrist extension, elbow extension, and shoulder abduction can help determine the condition of the posterior cord.

The latissimus dorsi is innervated by the thoracodorsal nerve, which is also a branch of the posterior cord. This area can be palpated in the posterior axillary fold and can be felt to contract when a patient is asked to cough, or to press his or her hands against his or her hip. The pectoralis major is innervated by the medial and lateral pectoral nerves, each a branch, respectively, of the medial and lateral cords. The lateral pectoral nerve innervates the clavicular head and the medial pectoral nerve innervates the sternal head of the pectoralis major. The entire pectoralis major can be palpated from superior to inferior as the patient adducts his or her arm against resistance.

Proximal to the cord level, the suprascapular nerve is a terminal branch at the trunk level. This area can be examined by assessing shoulder external rotation and elevation. Often in a chronic situation, the posterior aspect of the shoulder will show significant atrophy in the area of the infraspinatus muscle. Supraspinatus muscle atrophy is harder to detect clinically, because the trapezius muscle covers most of the muscle. The loss of shoulder flexion, rotation, and abduction can also

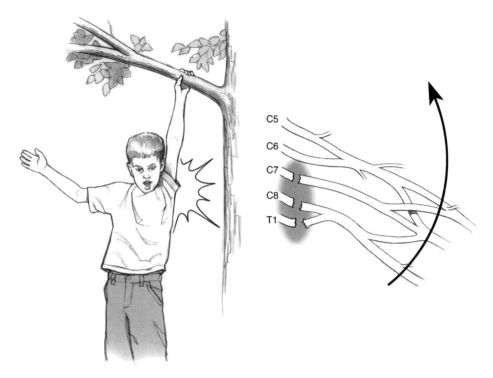

Fig. 7. With abduction and traction, as in a hanging injury, the lower elements of the plexus (C8, T1) can be injured. (Courtesy of the Mayo Foundation, Rochester, MN; with permission.)

be from a significant rotator cuff injury or deltoid injury. Axillary nerve function and rotator cuff integrity should be evaluated when testing shoulder function in addition to suprascapular nerve function.

Certain findings suggest preganglionic injury on clinical examination. For example, an injury to the long thoracic nerve or dorsal scapular nerve suggests a higher (more proximal) level of injury because both nerves originate at the root level (see Fig. 2). The long thoracic nerve is formed from the roots of C5-C7 and innervates the serratus anterior. The length of the nerve is more than 20 cm, and it is vulnerable to injury as it descends along the chest wall. Injury to this nerve with resultant serratus anterior dysfunction results in significant scapular winging as the patient attempts to forward elevate the arm. The dorsal scapular nerve is derived from C4-C5 and innervates the rhomboid muscles, often at a foraminal level. Careful examination will show atrophy of the rhomboids and parascapular muscles if this nerve is injured. The patient must be observed from the posterior to be able to fully evaluate the serratus anterior and rhomboid muscles.

Patients should also be examined for the presence of Horner's syndrome (Fig. 8). The sympathetic ganglion for T1 lies in close proximity to the T1 root and provides sympathetic outflow to the head and neck. The avulsion of the T1 root results in interruption of the T1 sympathetic ganglion and in Horner's syndrome, which consists of miosis (small pupil), enophthalmos (sinking of the orbit), ptosis (lid droop), and anhydrosis (dry eyes).

Motor testing must consider neighboring cranial nerves. For example, the spinal accessory nerve that innervates the trapezius muscle can occasionally be injured with neck or shoulder trauma that affects the brachial plexus. Its integrity is important because of the increasing use of the spinal accessory as a nerve transfer. Trapezial paralysis or partial paralysis results in a rotation of the scapula in addition to an inability to abduct the shoulder beyond 90°.

Careful sensory (or autonomic) examination should check various nerve distributions (especially autonomous zones). The sensation of root level dermatomes can be unreliable because of overlap from other nerves or anatomic variation.

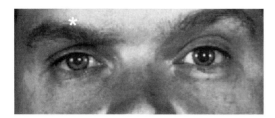

Fig. 8. Horner's syndrome. With avulsion of the left T1 root, the first thoracic sympathetic ganglion is injured. The result, shown on the patient's right side, is (*) miosis (constricted pupil), ptosis (drooped lid), anhydrosis (dry eyes), and enophthalmos (sinking of the eyeball). This patient showed miosis and ptosis after a lower trunk avulsion injury. (Courtesy of the Mayo Foundation, Rochester, MN; with permission.)

Active and passive range of motion should be recorded. Reflexes should be assessed. The physician should ensure that there is no evidence of concomitant spinal cord injury by examining for lower limb strength, sensory levels, increased reflexes, or pathologic reflexes. Percussing the nerve is especially helpful. Acutely, pain over a nerve suggests a rupture. An avulsion may be present when there is no percussion tenderness over the brachial plexus. An advancing Tinel's sign suggests a recovering lesion (as described previously).

A vascular examination should also be performed. This examination should include feeling distal pulses, feeling for thrills, or listening for bruits. It is possible to rupture the axillary artery in a significant brachial plexus injury. Vascular injuries are not an infrequent finding with infraclavicular lesions or with even more severe injuries, such as scapulothoracic dissociations, and should be evaluated and managed by a vascular surgeon either before or concomitantly with surgical intervention to the brachial plexus. In the acute setting, major concomitant injuries are present in 60% of patients, with most of these injuries being long bone fractures, followed by head injuries, chest injuries, and spinal fractures [9].

Radiographic evaluation

After a traumatic injury to the neck or shoulder girdle region, radiographic evaluation can give clues to the existence of associated neurologic injury. Standard radiographs should include cervical spine views, shoulder views (anteroposterior, axillary views), and a chest X ray. The cervical spine films should be examined for any associated cervical fractures, which could put the spinal cord at risk. In addition, the existence of transverse process fractures of the cervical vertebrae might indicate root avulsion at the same level. A fracture of the clavicle may also be an indicator of trauma to the brachial plexus. A chest X ray may show rib fractures (first or second ribs), suggesting damage to the overlying brachial plexus. Careful review of chest radiographs may give information regarding old rib fractures, which may become important should intercostal nerves be considered for nerve transfers (because rib fractures often injure the associated intercostal nerves). In addition, if the phrenic nerve is injured, there will be associated paralysis and elevation of the hemidiaphragm. Arteriography may be indicated in cases where vascular injury is suspected. Magnetic resonance angiography also may be useful to confirm the patency of a previous vascular repair or reconstruction.

CT combined with myelography has been instrumental in helping to define the level of nerve root injury [16,22,23]. When there is an avulsion of a cervical root, the dural sheath heals with development of a pseudomeningocele. Immediately after injury, a blood clot is often in the area of the nerve root avulsion and can displace dye from the myelogram. Therefore, a CT/myelogram should be performed 3 to 4 weeks after injury to allow time for any blood clots to dissipate and for pseudomeningocele to fully form. If a pseudomeningocele is seen on CT/myelogram, a root avulsion is likely (see Fig. 5).

MRI has improved over the past several years and can be helpful in evaluating the patient with a suspected nerve root avulsion [24–26]. It has some advantages over CT/myelogram because it is noninvasive and can visualize much of the brachial plexus, whereas CT/myelography shows only nerve root injury. MRI can reveal large neuromas after trauma and associated inflammation or edema. MRI of the brachial plexus can be helpful in evaluating mass lesions in the spontaneous nontraumatic neuropathy affecting the brachial plexus or its terminal branches. In acute trauma, however, CT/myelography remains the gold standard of radiographic evaluation for nerve root avulsion. MRI continues to improve, however, and may someday eliminate the need for the more invasive myelography.

Electrodiagnostic studies

Electrodiagnostic studies are an integral component of preoperative and intraoperative decision making when used appropriately and interpreted correctly. Electrodiagnostic studies can help confirm a diagnosis, localize lesions, define the severity of axon loss and the completeness of a lesion, eliminate other conditions from the differential diagnosis, and reveal subclinical recovery or unrecognized subclinical disorders. Electrodiagnostic studies therefore serve as an important adjunct to a thorough history, physical examination, and imaging studies, not as a substitute for them. When they are considered together, a decision can be made whether to proceed with operative intervention.

For closed injuries, baseline electromyography (EMG) and nerve conduction studies (NCSs) can best be performed 3 to 4 weeks after the injury because Wallerian degeneration will occur by this time. Serial electrodiagnostic studies can be performed in conjunction with a repeat physical examination every few months to document and quantify ongoing reinnervation or denervation.

EMG tests muscles at rest and with activity. Denervation changes (ie, fibrillation potentials) in different muscles can be seen in proximal muscles as early as 10 to 14 days after the injury and 3 to 6 weeks post injury in more distal muscles. Reduced motor unit potential (MUP) recruitment can be shown immediately after weakness from lower motor neuron injury occurs. The presence of active motor units with voluntary effort and few fibrillations at rest has a good prognosis compared with the absence of motor units and many fibrillations. EMG can help distinguish preganglionic from postganglionic lesions by needle examination of proximally innervated muscles that are innervated by root level motor branches (eg, cervical paraspinals, rhomboids, serratus anterior).

NCSs are also performed with the EMG. In post-traumatic brachial plexus lesions, the amplitudes of compound muscle action potentials (CMAPs) are generally low. SNAPs are important in localizing a lesion as preganglionic or postganglionic. SNAPs are preserved in lesions proximal to the DRG. Because the sensory nerve cell body is intact and within the DRG, NCSs will often show that the SNAP is normal and the motor conduction is absent, when clinically, the patient is insensate in the associated dermatome. SNAPs are absent in a postganglionic or combined pre- and postganglionic lesion. Because of overlapping sensory innervation, especially in the index finger, the physician needs to be cautious about the localization of the specific nerve with a preganglionic injury based on the SNAP alone.

There are obvious limitations to electrodiagnostic studies. The EMG/NCS is only as good as the experience of the physician in performing the study and interpreting the result. Certainly, EMG can show evidence of early recovery in muscles (ie, emergence of nascent potentials, a decreased number of fibrillation potentials, or the appearance or increased number of MUPs); these findings may predate clinically apparent recovery by weeks to months. EMG recovery does not always equate with clinically relevant recovery, however, either in terms of quality of regeneration or extent of recovery. It merely indicates that some unknown number of fibers has reached muscles and established motor end-plate connections. Conversely, EMG evidence of reinnervation may not be detected in complete lesions despite ongoing regeneration, when target end organs are further distal.

The current authors believe that intraoperative electrodiagnostic studies are a necessary part of brachial plexus surgery in helping guide decision making. They use a combination of intraoperative electrodiagnostic techniques to maximize the information gathered before making a surgical decision. They use nerve action potentials (NAPs) and somatosensory evoked potentials (SEPs) routinely, and occasionally use CMAPs. The use of NAPs allows a surgeon to test a nerve directly across a lesion, which allows the surgeon to detect reinnervation months before conventional EMG techniques and determine whether a lesion is neurapraxic (negative NAP) or axonotmetic (positive NAP). The presence of an NAP across a lesion indicates preserved axons or significant regeneration. Primate studies have suggested that the presence of an NAP indicates the viability of thousands of axons rather than hundreds as seen with other techniques [27]. The presence of an NAP bodes well for recovery after neurolysis alone, without the need for additional treatment (eg, neuroma resection and grafting). More than 90% of patients with a preserved NAP will gain clinically useful recovery. NAPs can indirectly help distinguish between pre- and postganglionic injury. A faster conduction velocity with large amplitude and short latency (with severe neurologic loss) indicates a preganglionic injury. A flat tracing suggests that adequate regeneration is not occurring; this finding would be consistent either with a postganglionic lesion that is reparable or a combined pre- and postganglionic lesion (irreparable). In the latter situation, sectioning the nerve back to an intraforaminal level would not reveal good fascicular structure [20].

Intraoperative SEPs are also used. The presence of an SEP suggests continuity between the peripheral nervous system and the central nervous system by means of a dorsal root. A positive response is determined by the integrity of few hundred intact fibers. The actual state of the ventral root is not tested directly by this technique; instead, it is inferred from the state of the sensory nerve rootlets, although there is not always perfect correlation between dorsal and ventral root avulsions. SEPs are absent in postganglionic or combined pre- and postganglionic lesions. Motor evoked potentials can assess the integrity of the motor pathway by means of the ventral root. This technique using transcranial electrical stimulation recently has been approved in the United States [28]. CMAPs are not useful in complete distal lesions because of the necessary time for regeneration to occur into distal muscles. CMAPs are useful in partial lesions where their size is proportional to the number of functioning axons. All of these techniques have limitations and technical challenges, but when performed with experienced neurologists or electrophysiologists, they can help guide treatment.

Summary

Most brachial plexus injuries involve the entire plexus. An injury to major cords or branches often contains a mixed injury pattern, with portions of the nerve being avulsed, ruptured, or stretched. An advancing Tinel's sign implies the possibility of neurologic recovery; however, the surgeon should combine this physical finding with that of electrodiagnostic studies to assess the extent of nerve injury to allow for expedient surgical intervention when necessary.

References

[1] Allieu Y, Cenac P. Is surgical intervention justifiable for total paralysis secondary to multiple avulsion injuries of the brachial plexus?. Hand Clin 1988; 4(4):609–18.

[2] Azze RJ, Mattar J Jr, Ferreira MC, Starck R, Canedo AC. Extraplexual neurotization of brachial plexus. Microsurgery 1994;15(1):28–32.

[3] Brandt KE, Mackinnon SE. A technique for maximizing biceps recovery in brachial plexus reconstruction. J Hand Surg 1993;18A(4):726–33.

[4] Brunelli G, Monini L. Direct muscular neurotization. J Hand Surg 1985;10A(6 Pt 2):993–7.

[5] Doi K, Muramatsu K, Hattori Y, et al. Restoration of prehension with the double free muscle technique

[6] Doi K, Kuwata N, Muramatsu K, Hottori Y, Kawai S. Double muscle transfer for upper extremity reconstruction following complete avulsion of the brachial plexus. Hand Clin 1999;15(4):757–67.

[7] Malone J, Leal J, Underwood J, et al. Brachial plexus injury management through upper extremity amputation with immediate postoperative prostheses. Arch Phys Med Rehabil 1982;63:89–91.

[8] Allieu Y. Evolution of our indications for neurotization. Our concept of functional restoration of the upper limb after brachial plexus injuries [in French]. Chir Main 1999;18(2):165–6.

[9] Dubuisson AS, Kline DG. Brachial plexus injury: a survey of 100 consecutive cases from a single service. Neurosurgery 2002;51(3):673–82 [discussion: 682–3].

[10] Narakas A. The treatment of brachial plexus injuries. Int Orthop 1985;9:29–36.

[11] Seddon HJ. Three types of nerve injury. Brain 1943; 66:238–88.

[12] Mackinnon SE. Nerve grafts. In: Goldwyn RM, Cohen MN, editors. The unfavorable result in plastic surgery. Philadelphia: Lippincott, Williams & Wilkins; 2001. p. 134–60.

[13] Narakas A, Bonnard C. Anatomopathological lesions. In: Alnot JY, Narakas A, editors. Traumatic brachial plexus injuries. Paris: Expansion Scientifique Francaise; 1996. p. 72–91.

[14] Songcharoen P, Shin AY. Brachial plexus injury: acute diagnosis and treatment. In: Berger RA, Weis APC, editors. Hand surgery. Philadelphia: Lippincott, Williams & Wilkins; 2004. p. 1005–25.

[15] Mackinnon SE, Dellon AL. Brachial plexus injuries. In: Mackinnon SE, Dellon AL, editors. Surgery of the peripheral nerve. New York: Thieme; 1988. p. 423–54.

[16] Nagano A, Ochiai N, Sugioka H, Hara T, Tsuyama N. Usefulness of myelography in brachial plexus injuries. J Hand Surg [Am] 1989;14B(1):59–64.

[17] Nagano A. Treatment of brachial plexus injury. J Orthop Sci 1998;3(1):71–80.

[18] Mansat M, Bonnevialle P. Mechanisms of traumatic plexus injuries. In: Alnot JY, Narakas A, editors. Traumatic brachial plexus injuries. Paris: Expansion Scientifique Francaise; 1996. p. 68–71.

[19] Horowitz SH. Brachial plexus injuries with causalgia resulting from transaxillary rib resection. Arch Surg 1985;120:1189–91.

[20] Sinow JD, Cunningham BL. Postmastectomy brachial plexus injury exacerbated by tissue expansion. Ann Plast Surg 1994;27:368–70.

[21] Luosto R, Ketonen P, Harjola PT, Jarvinen A. Extrathoracic approach for reconstruction of subclavian and vertebral arteries. Scand J Thorac Cardiovasc Surg 1980;14:227–31.

[22] Carvalho GA, Nikkhah G, Matthies C, Penkert G, Samii M. Diagnosis of root avulsions in traumatic

brachial plexus injuries: value of computerized tomography myelography and magnetic resonance
imaging. J Neurosurg 1997;86(1):69–76.

[23] Walker AT, Chaloupka JC, de Lotbiniere AC,
Wolfe SW, Goldman R, Kier EL. Detection of nerve
rootlet avulsion on CT myelography in patients with
birth palsy and brachial plexus injury after trauma.
AJR Am J Roentgenol 1996;167(5):1283–7.

[24] Doi K, Otsuka K, Okamoto Y, Fujii H, Hattori Y,
Baliarsing AS. Cervical nerve root avulsion in brachial plexus injuries: magnetic resonance imaging
classification and comparison with myelography
and computerized tomography myelography. J Neurosurg 2002;96(3 Suppl):277–84.

[25] Gupta RK, Mehta VS, Banerji AK, Jain RK. MR
evaluation of brachial plexus injuries. Neuroradiology 1989;31(5):377–81.

[26] Nakamura T, Yabe Y, Horiuchi Y, Takayama S.
Magnetic resonance myelography in brachial
plexus injury. J Bone Joint Surg [Br] 1997;79(5):
764–9.

[27] Tiel RL, Happel LT Jr, Kline DG. Nerve action potential recording method and equipment. Neurosurgery 1996;39(1):103–8.

[28] Burkholder LM, Houlden DA, Midha R, Weiss E,
Vennettilli M. Neurogenic motor evoked potentials:
role in brachial plexus surgery. Case report. J Neurosurg 2003;98(3):607–10.

ELSEVIER
SAUNDERS

Hand Clin 21 (2005) 25–37

HAND
CLINICS

Imaging the Brachial Plexus

Kimberly K. Amrami, MD[a],*, John D. Port, MD, PhD[b]

[a]Division of Body MRI, Department of Radiology, Mayo Clinic, 200 First Street SW, Rochester, MN 55905, USA
[b]Division of Neuroradiology, Department of Radiology, Mayo Clinic, 200 First Street SW, Rochester, MN 55905, USA

The brachial plexus is a network of nerves supplying sensory and motor innervation to the upper extremities extending from its origins from the C5 through T1 nerve roots laterally to the axilla. Clinically, evaluating lesions that involve the brachial plexus is challenging because of its inaccessibility to palpation and the complexity of its anatomy: the C5 and C6 rami form the upper trunk, the middle trunk arises from C7, and the lower trunk consists of the C8 and T1 rami. Each of these trunks divides into anterior and posterior divisions. They unite to form three cords, which are named relative to their relationship to the subclavian artery as follows: lateral (anterior divisions of the upper and middle trunks), posterior (posterior divisions of all three trunks), or medial (anterior division of the lower trunk). The cords divide into individual nerves, with their terminal branches as the musculocutaneous, median, axillary, radial, and ulnar nerves. The brachial plexus is surrounded by thoracic and axillary vascular structures, including the adjacent subclavian artery and vein, a large amount of fat, muscle, air in the lung, and the bony thorax and shoulder. In addition to this complex internal anatomy, there are many relatively acute angles where the neck and thorax join, creating multiple, abrupt air–tissue interfaces in the region of interest. This situation creates significant challenges for imaging this area. In general, a combination of high spatial resolution, multiplanar imaging capability, and good soft tissue contrast are required when considering lesions of the brachial plexus [1].

Multiple imaging modalities are available for evaluating the brachial plexus, the choice of which is highly dependent on the particular clinical circumstances. Plain-film myelography, postmyelography CT, MRI, ultrasound (US), and even positron emission tomography (PET) each have their place in imaging the brachial plexus. US has a relatively limited role, primarily because of its limited field of view and limitations in visualizing structures, such as bone and pleural abnormalities associated with tumor invasion [2]. Nerve disruption and vascular structures can be identified by a skilled practitioner and US may be used in some cases for guiding percutaneous intervention [2,3], but its role at this time is limited to those situations where MRI cannot be performed. MRI and post myelography CT are the mainstays of diagnosis of problems involving the brachial plexus. In general, abnormalities involving the brachial plexus can be divided into two broad categories for the purpose of imaging: traumatic and nontraumatic.

Traumatic brachial plexopathy

Overview

Traumatic brachial plexopathy, which accounts for approximately 50% of cases, can be caused by compression, stretching, or, in its most extreme form, disruption of nerves or avulsion of nerve roots, with or without fractures involving the cervical spine or clavicle [4]. If fracture is suspected, a radiograph (clavicle) or noncontrast CT with multiplanar reformatting (cervical spine) should be the initial study [4]. MRI is the study of choice for cases in which fractures of the clavicles or ribs may be causing extrinsic compression on the brachial plexus, typically the upper trunk

* Corresponding author.
E-mail address: amrami.kimberly@mayo.edu
(K.K. Amrami).

(Fig. 1), but suspected nerve root avulsion requires a different imaging algorithm.

The main cause of cervical and upper thoracic nerve root avulsion is a traction-induced injury, primarily from motorcycle accidents in adults [5] and shoulder dystocia in neonates. The prompt and accurate diagnosis of traumatic nerve root avulsions is essential to determine which patients might benefit from neurosurgical reconstruction. The prognosis and treatment options depend on differentiating preganglionic injuries from nerve

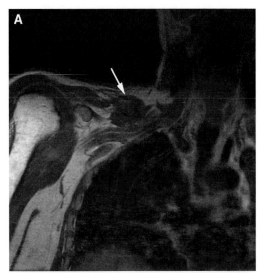

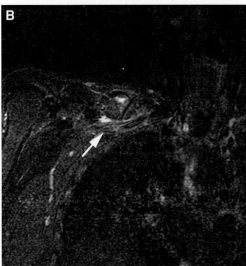

Fig. 1. Coronal T1 (*A*) and fat-suppressed FSE T2 (*B*) images of the right brachial plexus showing mass effect on the upper trunk from a displaced clavicle fracture (*arrow*). The upper trunk is enlarged and edematous.

root avulsion versus more distal postganglionic lesions from other causes [6].

Clinical examinations and electromyography (EMG) are occasionally inaccurate at determining the level or levels of the damaged roots because of normal anatomic variations within the brachial plexus [7–9]. The gold-standard test for determining nerve root avulsion remains the exploratory laminectomy, during which the surgeon directly evaluates the integrity of the dorsal and ventral nerve roots [10]. Because of the morbidity and mortality risks involved with such a procedure, few patients with suspected nerve root avulsions choose to undergo it.

Surgeons therefore have turned to neuroradiologic imaging procedures to determine the presence of nerve root avulsions. Traditional imaging modalities, such as radiography, MRI, and CT, have had mixed success in visualizing nerve roots; whereas these modalities are quite good at detecting the pseudomeningoceles associated with avulsions, reliably visualizing the nerve roots has been a persistent problem. Recent improvements in CT and MRI technology have made the reliable visualization of the roots possible on a routine clinical basis. These various imaging techniques are described in the following sections.

Plain-film myelography

With the advent of safe contrast agents for intrathecal injection, it became possible to detect nerve root avulsions using plain-film myelographic techniques. Several classic studies served as the foundation for noninvasive detection of cervical nerve root avulsion [11–13]. These plain-film techniques have become less important, however, because new CT methods provide better resolution and more accurate categorization of nerve root status. Therefore, these plain-film techniques will not be discussed further.

CT myelography

Early CT equipment, although revolutionary, suffered from many limitations, including large slice thicknesses. As a result, routine CT myelography was typically performed with a standard slice thickness of 5 mm, because that was the best the scanners could achieve at the time (eg, see references [14,15]). One study even concluded that plain-film myelography was more sensitive for detecting avulsions than CT myelography in the absence of pseudomeningocele [16]. These CT myelogram protocols still remain in common use

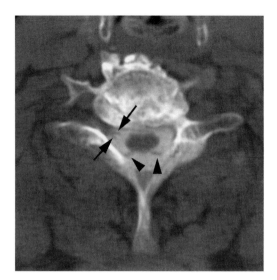

Fig. 2. Standard-resolution CT myelographic images (5 mm thick). Note that only the right exiting roots are visualized at this level (*arrows*); the left exiting roots are not seen. Also, because of the thickness of the slice, the dorsal roots for the adjacent level are also seen (*arrowheads*) but cannot be followed out to the neural foramina.

today. Although nerve roots are occasionally visualized using such thick slices, more often they are obscured because of partial volume artifacts, which render the roots undetectable. Fig. 2 shows a typical CT myelogram using a thickness of 5 mm; the roots are barely visible.

Because most cervical rootlets are approximately 1 mm thick, ideally they should be imaged with a 0.5-mm slice thickness to ensure adequate sampling (Nyquist limit, a basic rule of imaging physics). As the CT technology progresses, this theoretic possibility is becoming a reality. Currently available multidetector CT scanners can routinely scan with 1.25-mm slice thicknesses, and advanced 64-detector CT scanners will soon be available that can routinely scan slices as thin as 0.5 mm. Fig. 3 shows examples of partial and complete nerve root avulsions obtained using these thin-slice techniques. Two reconstruction algorithms are shown: a "hard-bone kernel" is used to preserve edge details at the expense of additional noise, whereas a "soft standard kernel" is used to reduce image noise at the expense of edge details. In the current authors' experience, hard kernels are more effective at detecting avulsions, because they accentuate the edges of the nerve roots relative to the adjacent myelogram dye.

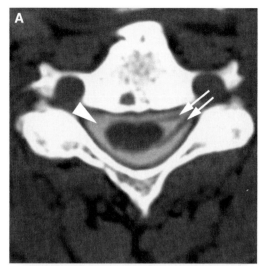

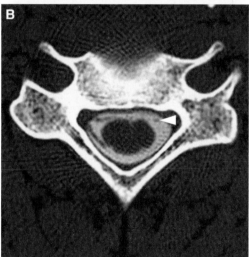

Fig. 3. High-resolution CT myelographic images (1.25 mm thick) of complete and partial nerve root avulsions. (*A*) Normal left dorsal and ventral roots (*arrows*) but complete avulsion of the right dorsal and ventral nerve roots (*arrowhead*) are shown. (*B*) Partial avulsion of the left ventral root (*arrowhead*). Note the thinning of the left ventral root relative to the right. The left dorsal root is completely avulsed. Note that (*A*) was reconstructed using soft kernels and (*B*) was reconstructed using a hard kernel. Image A therefore appears more blurry but less noisy than image B.

Realistically, no imaging technique is without artifacts. Occasionally, vessels in the thecal sac mimic nerve roots; a serpiginous vessel could easily be interpreted as a nerve root on static images. Likewise, scar tissue can occasionally mimic a nerve root, because the path of the scar tissue may be parallel to the nerve roots. Fig. 4 shows some of these pitfalls. In the authors' experience, by using the workstation to scroll through the image stack, in most cases we are able to visually trace the origin of the root from the cord and track it through the cerebrospinal fluid (CSF) into the neural foramen. Thus, even with high-quality source images, there can be difficulties confirming the presence of an avulsion.

Three-dimensional reconstructions may be helpful. Fig. 5 shows examples of complete nerve root avulsions as shown on coronal reconstructions performed using a postprocessing workstation. A curved-reformatting technique is used to "straighten" the cervical spine, allowing all the nerve roots to be visualized in a single slice. These reconstructions are labor-intensive, and require approximately 20 to 30 minutes for an experienced CT technologist to complete. Good reconstructions can be obtained; often, however, beam-hardening artifacts from the shoulders obscure details at the C7 and T1 levels, making interpretation difficult. Therefore, axial images are currently preferred for making determinations of nerve root avulsion.

MRI "myelography"

Magnetic resonance myelographic techniques are simply T2-weighted MRI sequences that accentuate the contrast between the spinal cord and roots and the adjacent CSF. These include regular spin-echo and fast spin-echo (FSE) techniques, and have various names depending on the particular MRI equipment vendor. Occasionally, gradient echo techniques are used, but these are less helpful because of reduced signal-to-noise ratios (SNRs) and lower native resolution.

Traditional MRI examinations also have suffered from partial volume artifacts; relatively thick slices are necessary to obtain acceptable SNRs at the expense of detecting the avulsions themselves. Furthermore, MRI also suffers from other artifacts, including patient motion (eg, swallowing, tremor, respiratory, cardiac) and CSF pulsation artifacts, which can also degrade image quality [17]. Fig. 6 shows some of these typical artifacts.

Several MRI studies have used axial 5-mm-thick slices, with variable success at detecting avulsions [18–24]. Others have tried oblique acquisitions in an attempt to minimize the effects of these artifacts. For example, Doi et al [25] used a thin-slice overlapping coronal oblique imaging

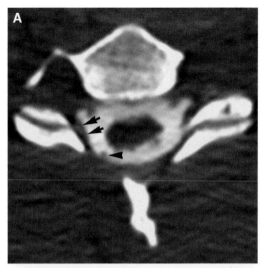

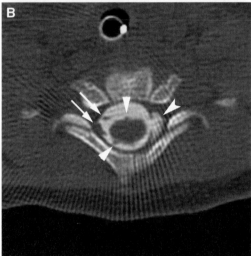

Fig. 4. High-resolution CT myelographic images (*A*, 1.25 mm thick; *B*, 0.675 mm thick, in a 5-month-old patient). (*A*) A linear density is shown lying on the posterolateral wall of the right neural foramen (*arrows*), presumably the right dorsal root. This "root" could not definitely be traced back to the cord, however, and therefore it probably represented scar tissue. The interpretation was further complicated by a small vessel (*arrowhead*), which touched the cord in a more rostral location, mimicking the origin of the right posterior root. (*B*) Several small vessels (*arrowheads*) are shown along the dorsal and ventral surface of the cord; these can occasionally be confused with nerve roots (*arrows*). The left dorsal and ventral roots are completely avulsed, although a root remnant is noted within the small left pseudomeningocele (*curved arrowhead*).

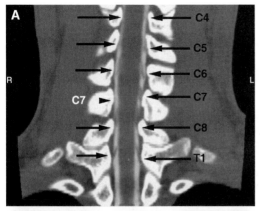

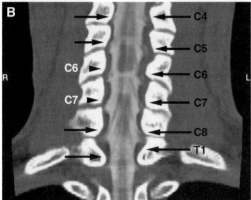

Fig. 5. Coronal reconstructions of high-resolution CT myelographic data sets. The cervical spine has been electronically "straightened" using a reformatting technique, such that all the dorsal and ventral roots are in a single plane. (*A*) All of the dorsal roots areshown in a single image (*arrows*). Note that the right C7 dorsal root is absent (*arrowhead*). (*B*) The ventral roots are shown in a single image (*arrows*). In this case, the right C6 and C7 roots (*arrowheads*) are absent. A small density is present in the expected location of the C6 root; this was believed to be scar tissue.

technique to better delineate the nerve roots. Although successful, the examination time was very long (25 min). In general, the thinner the MRI slice, the better the accuracy for detecting avulsions.

A relatively new MRI technique has recently become available called true fast imaging with steady-state precession (true-FISP), a variation of an older steady-state technique known as constructive interference in steady state (CISS). For an excellent outline of the history of true-FISP, see Gasparotti et al [6]. This technique generates good T2-weighted contrast with extremely thin slices while maintaining good SNR. The resulting

1- to 2-mm-thick slices are potentially quite useful for noninvasively evaluating nerve root avulsions [26]. Fig. 7 shows some images acquired with these techniques. As for all imaging techniques, however, these sequences are prone to artifact, with prominent "wrapping" artifacts contaminating the images at the edges of the image volume (eg, top and bottom slices for axial images). This is an active area of sequence development, and improvements should be commercially available within the next few years.

Nontraumatic brachial plexopathy

Overview

Nontraumatic brachial plexopathy may have a wide variety of causes, including the following: primary or metastatic tumors of neurogenic and other origins; inflammatory conditions, such as chronic inflammatory demyelinating polyneuropathy (CIDP) or brachial neuritis (Parsonage-Turner syndrome); or radiation fibrosis, commonly secondary to treatment for breast or lung cancer. For nontraumatic brachial plexopathy, MRI is the modality of choice for imaging [1,4,27]. The largest published review of brachial plexus imaging found that radiation fibrosis was the most common referral indication for the brachial plexus, but the range of pathology was broad, with breast and lung cancer far outweighing other primary and metastatic tumors, including lymphoma [28]. The current authors recently have witnessed an increase in requests for MRI of the brachial plexus in the evaluation of CIDP and its variants, primarily to localize signal abnormalities in the plexus for the purpose of biopsy and to follow up these patients during and after treatment. Neurogenic tumors and conditions, such as neurofibromatosis, are less commonly seen, but MRI is generally diagnostic for these entities because of their characteristic imaging features [2,27].

Patients may also present with nonspecific weakness or pain in the upper extremity, with or without EMG evidence of brachial plexopathy. In this instance, MRI is helpful to localize any suspected or unsuspected pathology, such as a mass, and to exclude any structural cause for the patient's symptoms.

Nonmyelographic MRI

Conventional, or nonmyelographic, MRI of the brachial plexus is the study of choice for nontraumatic brachial plexopathy because of its

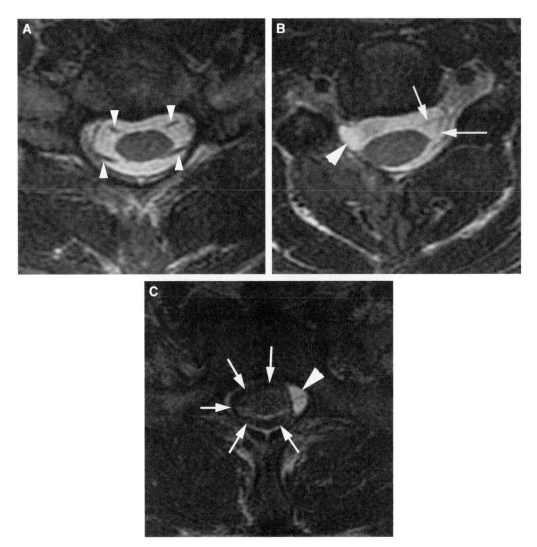

Fig. 6. Traditional FSE T2-weighted cervical spine MR images (TR = 2800, TE = 105, NEX = 3, slice 4 mm skip 0 mm, 384 × 256 matrix). (*A*) Occasionally, traditional images show nerve roots quite clearly (*arrowheads*). (*B*) More often, however, the MRI only vaguely suggests the presence of nerve roots (*arrows*). In this patient, the right dorsal and ventral roots are not visualized (*arrowhead*), but the physician cannot be certain if they are truly present or absent. (*C*) If a patient has prominent CSF pulsation artifact (*arrows*), nerve roots are not visible. Note that, in this case, the small pseudomeningocele (*arrowhead*) shows no flow artifact, therefore demonstrating the small root remnant. NEX, number of excitations; TE, time to echo; TR, time to repetition.

superior tissue contrast when compared with CT and US. Its multiplanar capability and ability to separate vascular and nonvascular structures from surrounding soft tissue, with or without the use of intravenous contrast material, are helpful adjuncts to treatment and surgical planning. As mentioned previously, however, achieving an artifact-free MRI examination of the brachial plexus is nearly impossible because of the combination of respiratory motion, vascular and CSF pulsation, and

susceptibility artifacts created by the abrupt air–tissue interfaces at the junction of the neck and trunk and the soft tissues of the neck and air in the lung. Because of these issues, meticulous attention must be paid to technique to optimize MRI examinations of the brachial plexus.

Low-field systems (<1.5 T) are of limited value in evaluating the brachial plexus. Conventional (1.5 T) and high-field (>3.0 T) imaging systems are required to achieve the optimal SNR and

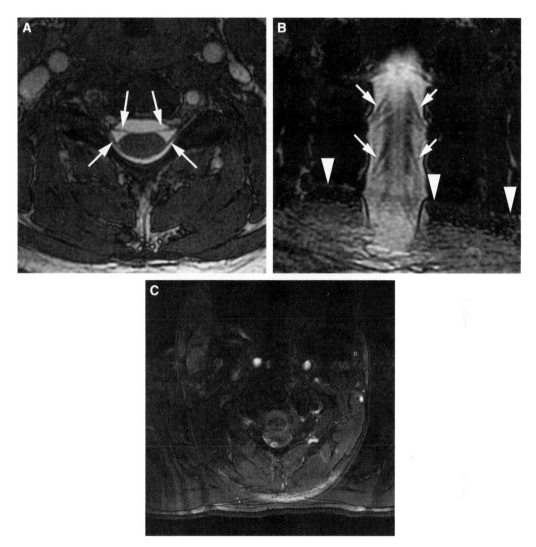

Fig. 7. New CISS T2-weighted cervical spine MR images (GE phase cycle FIESTA [GE Medical Systems, Milwaukee, Wisconsin], TR = 5.6, TE = 2.5, NEX = 2, flip angle 25, slice 1.5 mm skip 0 mm, 512 × 512 matrix). (*A*) There is good visualization of the nerve roots (*arrows*) throughout most of the scanned region. (*B*) Multiplanar imaging is also possible. This coronal image shows several ventral roots (*arrows*), although because of the normal curvature of the cervical spine, only a few ventral roots are visible in any given slice. Note also the prominent "wrap-around" artifact (*arrowheads*) from the fat of the back that obscures some image detail. (*C*) More prominent wrap-around artifact, with signal from the head contaminating the upper thoracic spine slices, renders these images uninterpretable. NEX, number of excitations; TE, time to echo; TR, time to repetition.

contrast-to-noise ratio necessary for these examinations. Moderate- to high-performing gradient systems are desirable for faster imaging sequences, including breath-hold and steady-state sequences, such as the true-FISP mentioned previously. Magnetic field homogeneity should be optimized on any system but is particularly important for these examinations, because fat saturation is recommended for both T2-weighted and

postcontrast imaging. High spatial resolution T2-weighted imaging with fat suppression, sometimes referred to as "MR neurography," is particularly important for identifying subtle signal changes within the individual nerves of the brachial plexus.

Dedicated surface coils are an important element of successful imaging of the brachial plexus [1]. Standard neurovascular coils provide high

SNR but rarely extend laterally to include the entire brachial plexus. The body coil is often used in clinical practice for brachial plexus examinations but provides limited SNR and makes achieving in-plane resolution and thin sections (≤4 mm) difficult. Torso or cardiac arrays may be used, offset to the side of interest. The ideal brachial plexus coil would incorporate elements of the neurovascular and torso arrays but is not available except where custom-made for individual practices. Recently, vendors have been offering a combination of coils that create panoramic coverage; this use of a flexible combination of coil elements for brachial plexus coverage seems promising, but clinical experience is lacking. A surface coil, even if somewhat awkward for placement, is superior to the use of the body coil for all brachial plexus MRI.

High-field (≥3.0 T) imaging of the brachial plexus provides some distinct advantages, the most important of which is the overall increase in signal, which allows for improved spatial resolution without a significant increase in background noise when compared with studies performed at 1.5 T. This advantage translates into improved detail and sharper images for detecting subtle changes in signal intensity or morphology in the brachial plexus. A further benefit is the improved field strength–dependent chemical fat suppression, which allows for the consistent use of spin-echo (conventional and fast), T2-weighted, fat-suppressed sequences with high intrinsic SNR rather than relying on inversion recovery techniques. These techniques, such as short tau inversion recovery (STIR) and FSE inversion recovery (FSEIR), rely on the application of inversion pulses, imaging on the null point of fat. Although the fat saturation is robust, these sequences are relatively signal poor and pulsation artifacts are accentuated, which can obscure pathology within the plexus (Fig. 8). If higher order shim is not available at conventional field strengths, inversion recovery techniques can provide good T2-weighted imaging with fat suppression that does not depend on magnetic field homogeneity. Breath-hold pulse sequences, such as fast recovery FSE, single-shot FSE, and others, have tried to overcome some of the intrinsic problems with brachial plexus imaging. Generally, however, the T2 contrast has not been adequate to distinguish subtle signal changes. True-FISP, or FIESTA (fast imaging employing steady-state acquisition), provides very high spatial resolution and thin sections with both two- and three-dimensional modes, with acceptable T2

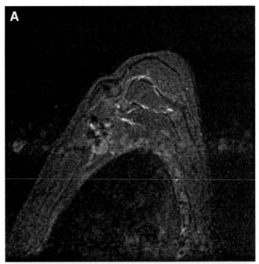

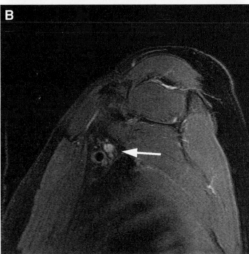

Fig. 8. Sagittal STIR image of the infraclavicular brachial plexus (*A*) shows significant pulsation and respiratory artifacts. FSE T2 with fat suppression (*B*) clearly shows thickening and abnormal signal in the posterior cord of the brachial plexus (*arrow*). This patient had severe triceps weakness. Biopsy showed perineurinoma involving the posterior cord and radial nerve.

contrast, but the phase artifacts particular to that sequence and the lack of fat suppression currently limit its application on a routine basis (see Fig. 7).

Images should be obtained in axial, sagittal, and coronal planes with both T1 and fat-suppressed T2 weighting. The authors offset images to the side of interest to optimize spatial resolution, with the exception of the axial plane when a bilateral examination is requested. Their basic protocol includes an FSE T1-weighted axial sequence, parasagittal images through the brachial plexus from lateral to medial using both T1-weighted and fat-suppressed T2-weighted images (both typically FSE), and an oblique coronal plane that shows most of the plexus laid out from its origin to the axilla. This last group of images is prescribed from a sagittal image in the region of the infraclavicular brachial plexus. The slice thickness and field of view should be as small as possible to maximize spatial resolution. The authors typically use a field of view of 22 cm, with slice thickness of 4 to 5 mm and acquisition matrix of more than 256. If contrast material is administered, it is important for postcontrast images to be fat suppressed. The authors use either fat-suppressed T1-weighted spin-echo or T1-weighted, two-dimensional spoiled gradient recalled echo imaging in at least two places. If angiographic images are desired for surgical planning, a magnetic resonance angiogram (MRA) can be performed using three-dimensional time-of-flight techniques with real-time bolus tracking to optimize the visualization of thoracic and axillary vessels. Slightly delayed postcontrast static images can then be performed without any compromise of image quality. Total imaging time, even with an MRA, is usually less than 45 minutes for a unilateral examination.

MRI is the study of choice for characterizing and distinguishing the cause of nontraumatic brachial plexopathies [28]. The following sections discuss some of the more common entities involving the brachial plexus and their appearance on MRI.

Common causes of nontraumatic brachial plexopathy

Radiation fibrosis

Radiation fibrosis is a common sequela of the external beam radiotherapy used to treat tumors such as breast cancer and lung cancer. Patients may present with symptoms of nerve damage as early as 5 months and up to approximately 3 years after treatment, with the peak incidence of symptoms occurring between 10 and 20 months. The degree of damage is dose-dependent, with higher doses resulting in greater disability. In general, if symptoms, such as painless weakness, present in the first year after treatment, radiation damage is more likely to be the cause than is tumor recurrence [4]. MRI findings of radiation fibrosis include diffuse thickening and enhancement of the brachial plexus without a discrete mass [27,28]. In general, signal intensity is low on both T1- and T2-weighted imaging, which may help to distinguish radiation fibrosis from tumor recurrence. Increased signal on T2 weighting may help to differentiate tumor from fibrosis, but this finding is not sensitive or specific enough to be a reliable sign [29]. In late cases (>5 y after treatment), these differences may be more helpful in distinguishing recurrent tumor or a late sequela of treatment, such as lymphoma.

Inflammatory brachial plexopathy

CIDP is probably an immune-mediated neuropathy, which is characterized histologically by recurrent demyelination, remyelination, and inflammation [4]. MRI findings, when this condition involves the brachial plexus, include hypertrophy of the nerves of the brachial plexus, with mild to moderate increased T2 signal. Enhancement is not a feature of this entity. MRI is useful for confirming and localizing abnormality in conjunction with EMG and to exclude mass lesions, which may cause similar symptoms. Treatments such as immunoglobulins and plasmapharesis may be effective, and MRI can be used to monitor changes in signal intensity in the nerves over time.

Brachial neuritis (Parsonage-Turner syndrome) is a syndrome characterized by shoulder girdle weakness and pain of acute onset. The cause of the disorder is not known, but antecedent viral or other infections are commonly identified in sufferers. MRI may show increased T2 signal in the nerves and edema and even atrophy in the muscles of the shoulder girdle, but without discrete nerve thickening or masses [4,28]. Soft tissue edema may be present around the plexus as a sign of inflammation. The imaging findings of brachial neuritis are, however, nonspecific, and the diagnosis is primarily one of exclusion.

Breast and lung cancer

Primary lung cancers arising at the apex of the lung, commonly called Pancoast's tumors, have a propensity to extend beyond the lung into the soft tissues of the neck, including the brachial plexus. The syndrome associated with these tumors includes pain in the C8 and T1 distribution, muscle atrophy of the hand, and Horner's syndrome in approximately 20% of cases [4,27]. MRI is the preferred modality for identifying both the primary tumor and the specific site of tumor invasion (Fig. 9) in the brachial plexus.

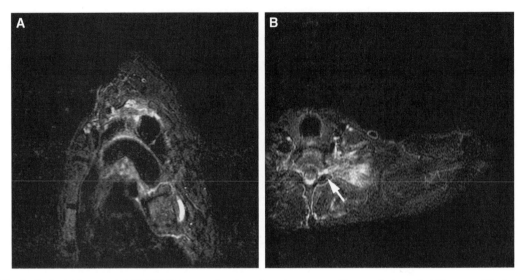

Fig. 9. Sagittal (*A*) and axial (*B*) FSEIR images showing a large lung cancer (Pancoast's tumor) at the apex of the lung. The tumor is invading the lower trunk of the brachial plexus, extending into the C8 foramen (*arrow*). The patient presented with arm weakness and pain, which improved after radiation to the area.

Metastatic lymphadenopathy of the axilla and supraclavicular region is frequent in breast cancer because of the major lymphatic drainage of the breast through the apex of the axilla [27]. In addition, metastasis may directly invade the brachial plexus causing pain and other neurologic symptoms, such as weakness. As discussed previously, presentation of these symptoms in the first year is usually because of direct damage from radiotherapy, but the appearance of these symptoms 5, 10, or even 15 years later is an ominous sign and likely because of tumor recurrence [30]. Recurrent tumor may present as discrete masses or as infiltration along the nerve of

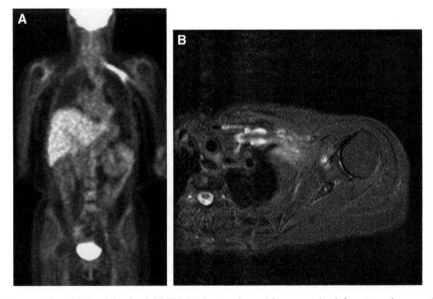

Fig. 10. PET scan (*A*) and T2-weighted axial MRI (*B*) in a patient with progressive left-arm weakness and pain with a remote (20 y prior) history of breast cancer. The avid uptake on the PET scan and increased T2 signal on MRI distinguishes the patient's recurrent breast cancer from radiation fibrosis.

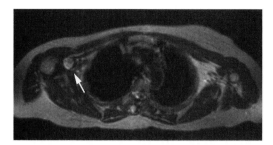

Fig. 11. Axial T2-weighted spin-echo image of a mass (*arrow*) in the right brachial plexus showing the "target" sign typical of neurogenic tumors. This mass was excised and shown to be a schwannoma.

the plexus. In the latter case, it may be impossible to distinguish the imaging changes from nonspecific inflammatory or other processes. A high level of suspicion and the use of adjunct imaging tools, such as PET (Fig. 10), may be needed to accurately diagnose late recurrence.

Neurogenic tumors

Approximately 20% of all tumors of peripheral nerves arise in the brachial plexus [2,31]. Schwannomas, neurofibromas, and malignant peripheral nerve sheath tumors (MPNSTs) may occur there, with neurofibromas being the most common [4]. One third of neurofibromas occur in patients with neurofibromatosis type 1, and these lesions are usually multiple. The imaging features of solitary neurofibromas overlap those of schwannomas,

with ovoid shapes, T1 signal intensity isointense to muscle, and very bright T2 signal, usually with avid contrast enhancement. Benign neurogenic tumors have a characteristic appearance on T2-weighted imaging, which has been referred to as a "target" sign—a central area of decreased T2 signal believed to represent organized collagen fibers (Fig. 11). MPNSTs recently have been reported to be distinguishable from benign tumors on MRI by their size, irregularity, and areas of nonenhancing necrosis after contrast administration, but there is too much overlap between these entities to reliably make this distinction with imaging alone [31]. Rapid growth in a mass suggests malignancy but often only biopsy can provide an accurate diagnosis.

Other tumors and tumorlike conditions may involve the brachial plexus, including benign lipomas, aggressive fibromatosis, lymphoma, metastases from other primary tumors, such as melanoma, and even Ewing's sarcoma spreading from the adjacent clavicle in children [28]. An unusual entity called perineurinoma, or localized hypertrophic neuropathy, typically involves a single peripheral nerve and results in progressive weakness in a specific neural distribution. On MRI, these may appear as fusiform areas of thickening, which may mimic a neoplastic process (Fig. 12). Fibrolipomatous hamartoma is a very rare, benign, infiltrating condition involving peripheral nerves, most commonly the median and sciatic nerves. A single case has been reported in the brachial plexus [32]. MRI

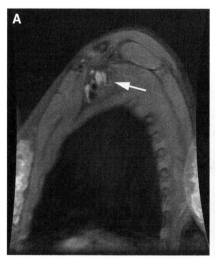
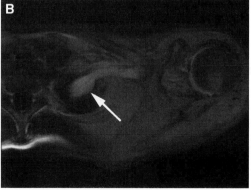

Fig. 12. Sagittal (*A*) and axial (*B*) T2-weighted images of the brachial plexus in a 12-year-old girl with hand weakness. There is fusiform enlargement (*arrow*) of the middle trunk. Biopsy showed a perineurinoma.

of this entity has a characteristic appearance, with fusiform enlargement of the nerve with fatty proliferation within the nerve itself.

Summary

Imaging the brachial plexus is challenging because of the complex anatomy of the region and the wide variety of pathology that can affect it. For the purpose of imaging, it is helpful to divide traumatic and nontraumatic entities affecting the brachial plexus. Improvements in imaging technology, including multidetector CT for CT myelography and the availability of full-field-strength MRI systems with fast gradients and dedicated surface coils for optimal spatial resolution, have led to more accurate prospective diagnoses and improved aid for neurosurgical planning for traumatic and nontraumatic brachial plexopathies. CT myelography is the current gold standard for the diagnosis of nerve root avulsions affecting the brachial plexus. MRI is the preferred modality for nontraumatic brachial plexopathy. Other modalities, such as US and PET, have a limited role in the evaluation of brachial plexus pathology. High-quality, high-resolution CT and MRI remain the mainstays for imaging the brachial plexus.

References

[1] Qayyum A, MacVicar AD, Padhani AR, Revell P, Husband JE. Symptomatic brachial plexopathy following treatment for breast cancer: utility of MR imaging with surface-coil techniques. Radiology 2000; 214(3):837–42.

[2] Rettenbacher T, Sogner P, Springer P, Fiegl M, Hussl H, zur Nedden D. Schwannoma of the brachial plexus: cross-sectional imaging diagnosis using CT, sonography, and MR imaging. Eur Radiol 2003; 13(8):1872–5.

[3] Graif M, Martinoli S, Rochkind S. Sonographic evaluation of brachial plexus pathology. Eur Radiol 2004;14:193–200.

[4] Hyodoh K, Hyodoh H, Akiba H, et al. Brachial plexus: normal anatomy and pathological conditions. Curr Probl Diagn Radiol 2002;31(5):179–88.

[5] Goldie BS, Coates CJ. Brachial plexus injury: a survey of incidence and referral pattern. J Hand Surg [Br] 1992;17(1):86–8.

[6] Gasparotti R, Ferraresi S, Pinelli L, et al. Three-dimensional MR myelography of traumatic injuries of the brachial plexus. AJNR Am J Neuroradiol 1997;18(9):1733–42.

[7] Miller R. Observations upon the arrangement of the axillary and brachial plexus. Am J Anat 1939;64:143.

[8] Kerr A. Brachial plexus of nerves in man. The variations in its formation and branches. Am J Anat 1918; 23:285–395.

[9] Sherman WL, Hays AP, Lange DJ, Latov N, Trojaborg W, Younger DS. Clinical, electrophysiological, and myelographic studies of 9 patients with cervical spinal root avulsions: discrepancies between EMG and X-ray findings. Neurology 1995;45(4):827–9.

[10] Oberle J, Antoniadis G, Rath SA, et al. Radiological investigations and intra-operative evoked potentials for the diagnosis of nerve root avulsion: evaluation of both modalities by intradural root inspection. Acta Neurochir [Wien] 1998;140(6):527–31.

[11] Cobby MJ, Leslie IJ, Watt I. Cervical myelography of nerve root avulsion injuries using water-soluble contrast media. Br J Radiol 1988;61(728):673–8.

[12] Nagano A, Ochiai N, Sugioka H, Hara T, Tsuyama N. Usefulness of myelography in brachial plexus injuries. J Hand Surg [Br] 1989;14(1):59–64.

[13] Yeoman PM. Cervical myelography in traction injuries of the brachial plexus. J Bone Joint Surg [Br] 1968;50(2):253–60.

[14] Petras AF, Sobel DF, Mani JR, Lucas PR. CT myelography in cervical nerve root avulsion. J Comput Assist Tomogr 1985;9(2):275–9.

[15] Morris RE, Hasso AN, Thompson JR, Hinshaw DB Jr, Vu LH. Traumatic dural tears: CT diagnosis using metrizamide. Radiology 1984;152(2):443–6.

[16] Hashimoto T, Mitomo M, Hirabuki N, et al. Nerve root avulsion of birth palsy: comparison of myelography with CT myelography and somatosensory evoked potential. Radiology 1991;178(3):841–5.

[17] Volle E, Assheuer J, Hedde JP, Gustorf-Aeckerle R. Radicular avulsion resulting from spinal injury: assessment of diagnostic modalities. Neuroradiology 1992;34(3):235–40.

[18] Vielvoye GJ, Hoffmann CF. Neuroradiological investigations in cervical root avulsion. Clin Neurol Neurosurg 1993;95(Suppl):S36–8.

[19] Francel PC, Koby M, Park TS, et al. Fast spin-echo magnetic resonance imaging for radiological assessment of neonatal brachial plexus injury. J Neurosurg 1995;83(3):461–6.

[20] Ochi M, Ikuta Y, Watanabe M, Kimori K, Itoh K. The diagnostic value of MRI in traumatic brachial plexus injury. J Hand Surg [Br] 1994;19(1):55–9.

[21] Gupta RK, Mehta VS, Banerji AK, Jain RK. MR evaluation of brachial plexus injuries. Neuroradiology 1989;31(5):377–81.

[22] Rapoport S, Blair DN, McCarthy SM, Desser TS, Hammers LW, Sostman HD. Brachial plexus: correlation of MR imaging with CT and pathologic findings. Radiology 1988;167(1):161–5.

[23] Roger B, Travers V, Laval-Jeantet M. Imaging of posttraumatic brachial plexus injury. Clin Orthop Rel Res 1988;(237):57–61.

[24] Nakamura T, Yabe Y, Horiuchi Y, Takayama S. Magnetic resonance myelography in brachial plexus injury. J Bone Joint Surg [Br] 1997;79(5):764–9.

[25] Doi K, Otsuka K, Okamoto Y, Fujii H, Hattori Y, Baliarsing AS. Cervical nerve root avulsion in brachial plexus injuries: magnetic resonance imaging classification and comparison with myelography and computerized tomography myelography. J Neurosurg 2002;96(3 Suppl):277–84.

[26] Baskaran V, Pereles FS, Russell EJ, et al. Myelographic MR imaging of the cervical spine with a 3D true fast imaging with steady-state precession technique: initial experience. Radiology 2003;227(2): 585–92.

[27] Kichari JR, Hussain SM, Den Hollander JC, Krestin GP. MR imaging of the brachial plexus: current imaging sequences, normal findings, and findings in a spectrum of focal lesions with MR-pathologic correlation. Curr Probl Diagn Radiol 2003;32(2): 88–101.

[28] Wittenberg KH, Adkins MC. MR imaging of nontraumatic brachial plexopathies: frequency and spectrum of findings. Radiographics 2000;20(4): 1023–32.

[29] Lingawi SS, Bilbey JH, Munk PL, et al. MR imaging of brachial plexopathy in breast cancer patients without palpable recurrence. Skeletal Radiol 1999; 28(6):318–23.

[30] Zingale A, Ponzo G, Ciavola G, Vagnoni G. Metastatic breast cancer delayed brachial plexopathy. A brief case report. J Neurosurg Sci 2002;46(3–4): 147–9.

[31] Saifuddin A. Imaging tumours of the brachial plexus. Skeletal Radiol 2003;32(7):375–87.

[32] Lai PH, Ho JT, Lin SL, et al. Neuromuscular hamartoma arising in the brachial plexus. Neuroradiology 2004;46(3):216–8.

ELSEVIER
SAUNDERS

Hand Clin 21 (2005) 39–46

HAND
CLINICS

Preoperative and Intraoperative Electrophysiologic Assessment of Brachial Plexus Injuries

C. Michel Harper, MD

Mayo Clinic, Mayo Clinic College of Medicine, 200 First Street SW, Rochester, MN 55905, USA

Nerve conduction studies (NCSs) and needle electromyography (EMG) are extensions of the neurologic examination that allow the examiner to study the physiology of healthy and diseased components of the peripheral nervous system (PNS). The PNS is organized into motor, sensory, and autonomic units. The motor unit consists of all muscle fibers innervated by the terminal branches of a single alpha motor neuron. The sensory unit is represented by the terminal end-organ branches and receptors connected to a single dorsal root ganglion (DRG) cell. The autonomic unit is composed of pre- and postganglionic neurons that synapse in ganglia associated with craniosacral (parasympathetic) or thoracolumbar (sympathetic) spinal segments. The study of autonomic physiology requires special techniques, which are not discussed in this article. The motor unit is studied with motor NCSs, needle EMG, and specialized techniques, such as motor evoked potentials (MEPs). The sensory unit is studied with sensory NCSs and somatosensory evoked potentials (SEPs).

Preoperative electrodiagnosis

NCSs and needle EMG are the primary studies used to gain information on the location, number, and pathophysiology of lesions affecting the brachial plexus and other peripheral nerves before surgical exploration. NCSs are often accurate enough to localize lesions within several centimeters along the course of a nerve segment. In motor NCSs, a mixed or pure motor nerve is stimulated at several places along the nerve. The

summated electrical response of all muscle fibers innervated by the activated axons (typically recorded with surface electrodes) is called the compound muscle action potential (CMAP). The size of the CMAP recorded after supramaximal stimulation of the peripheral nerve is directly related to the number of functioning motor axons. The size of the CMAP quantifies the number of activated axons, whereas the conduction velocity and distal latency measure conduction along the course of the motor axons.

To properly localize a lesion with motor NCSs, the physician must stimulate the nerve or fascicles of interest in isolation from other nearby nerves, or isolate the recording to muscle fibers innervated exclusively by the nerve or fascicles of interest. Another important criterion for localizing lesions involves stimulation or recording "through" the lesion. Stimulating or recording above and below the involved segment should isolate the segment of nerve that contains the lesion.

Sensory conduction studies involve the stimulation and recording of mixed or cutaneous nerves at one or more locations, recording the triphasic sensory nerve action potential (SNAP) at another location along the nerve. The SNAP represents summated action potentials of sensory axons. Thus, the SNAP has a lower amplitude, shorter duration, and different configuration (triphasic versus biphasic) than the CMAP (Fig. 1). These characteristics make the SNAP more difficult to record under "noisy" conditions.

The sensory neuron is unique in that the cell body is located outside the spinal cord in the DRG, which creates a pre- and postganglionic portion of the peripheral sensory axon (Fig. 2). When the lesion affects the preganglionic portion

E-mail address: mharper@mayo.edu

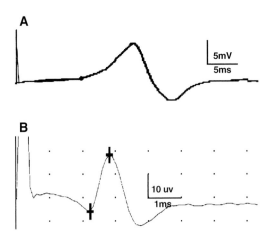

Fig. 1. (*A*) CMAP recording. Note the biphasic appearance, large amplitude, and long duration of the potential. (*B*) SNAP recording. Note the triphasic appearance, small amplitude, and short duration of the potential.

(between the DRG and spinal cord), the postganglionic axon remains in continuity with the DRG cell body, thus retaining its electrical excitability. In contrast, when the lesion is distal to the DRG (postganglionic), Wallerian degeneration occurs and the distal segment becomes electrically inexcitable. This phenomenon can be used to help localize lesions within the PNS. In the setting of a clinical sensory loss, the preservation of the SNAP in the distribution of the sensory loss indicates pathology proximal to the DRG (Fig. 3), whereas pathology distal to the DRG will reduce the amplitude of the SNAP in proportion to the severity of sensory axon loss.

Needle EMG is used to examine the characteristics of individual or groups of motor units within individual muscles. A loss of functioning motor

units is represented by reduced recruitment, where few motor unit potentials (MUPs) are present but discharge at faster frequencies in an attempt to maintain force production. Reduced recruitment is the hallmark of lower motor neuron or PNS weakness and is differentiated from poor activation, which occurs in weakness of central nervous system origin (or is from poor effort caused by pain, hysteria, or malingering). Reduced MUP recruitment is present as soon as weakness of lower motor neurons develops. There is no time delay. After 10 to 21 days, denervated muscle fibers begin to discharge under the influence of their intrinsic pacemaker (fibrillation potentials), and MUP begin to become polyphasic and enlarge (increase in duration and amplitude).

The exact findings on needle EMG depend on the severity and completeness of injury, the distance from the site of injury to the involved muscle, the time since the injury has occurred, and the progress and mechanism of regeneration. If a muscle has fibrillation potentials or MUP changes suggesting denervation and reinnervation, then there is a lesion at or proximal to the nerve branch to that muscle. Because of the fascicular anatomy of nerves, the converse cannot be stated as true. That is, if the muscle is normal, the lesion may still be proximal to the branch to that muscle. This occurrence is frequent in focal neuropathies and represents one of the main limitations of relying too heavily on localization based on needle EMG findings alone.

The application of NCSs and needle EMG to the study of complicated focal neuropathies, such as brachial plexus injuries, can provide useful information, but there are also limitations of these techniques performed in the preoperative setting. In severe plexopathies with a flail anesthetic arm, the presence of well-defined SNAPs in the

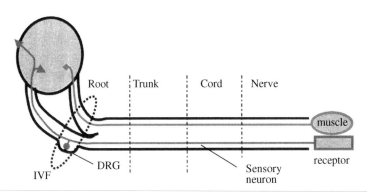

Fig. 2. Sensory and motor pathways. IVF, intervertebral foramen.

distribution of all spinal segments (C5–T1) indicates complete root avulsion at all levels. In less severe plexopathies, general segmental (C5–T1) and longitudinal (trunk, cord, nerve) localization is possible in most cases.

The presence of partial lesions with residual innervation or ongoing collateral reinnervation of muscles can be confirmed with either NCSs or needle EMG. The severity of axon loss in partial lesions can be defined in most cases on preoperative studies. Fibrillation potentials in paraspinal muscles indicate at least partial root injury in at least one cervical spinal segment.

Improvement associated with reinnervation can be documented and quantified on serial examinations.

In severe plexopathies with a flail anesthetic arm, the absence of SNAPs indicates damage to postganglionic elements but does not exclude a mixed lesion with associated root avulsion. Thus, one limitation of preoperative studies is the inability to detect root avulsion in the setting of a severe coexisting postganglionic injury. In addition, because of overlapping innervation, the presence of fibrillation potentials at multiple cervical paraspinal levels does not exclude the possibility that some cervical roots are intact.

The precise segmental and longitudinal location of partial and complete lesions of postganglionic elements is also limited in many patients with complex brachial plexus injuries because of difficulties in stimulating and recording affected fascicles in isolation and difficulties stimulating areas proximal and distal to the lesioned segments. Needle EMG is also limited by false localization because of selective fascicular involvement and because early regeneration cannot be detected

in complete lesions before the regenerating fibers reach their target muscle.

Intraoperative electrodiagnosis

Many of the limitations of preoperative electrodiagnosis are overcome by performing similar studies on exposed nerves during brachial plexus reconstruction. In this setting, electrophysiologic studies provide additional information about the number, location, type, and severity of nerve lesions [1,2]. This information can be used to answer important questions left unresolved by preoperative electrodiagnostic studies and to help surgeons make important therapeutic decisions regarding decompression, neurolysis, grafting, or neurotization of nerves [3]. With minor modifications, standard techniques of electrodiagnosis, such as NCS, EMG, and SEPs, are used to monitor the PNS during surgery. [2,4] Appropriate monitoring protocols can be designed for each patient after the findings of the preoperative neurologic examination, NCS, EMG, and surgical goals are reviewed.

Intraoperative techniques

Stimulation

A handheld bipolar electrical stimulator is placed directly onto the nerve within the surgical field (Fig. 4). The size of the stimulator is matched to the size of nerve. Larger stimulators similar to those used in routine NCSs are used to stimulate large nerve trunks that are isolated from other nerves. Hooked stimulating electrodes can be used to elevate nerves or fascicles from surrounding tissue when better stimulus isolation is required. Small electrodes are used when individual or small groups of fascicles are stimulated.

Intraoperative stimulation requires careful consideration of the location and strength of stimulus. Normal nerves are activated with as little

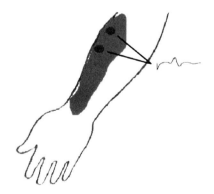

Fig. 3. Preserved SNAP in area of sensory loss indicates preganglionic pathology in brachial plexus lesions.

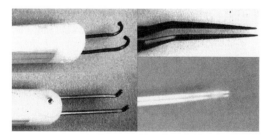

Fig. 4. Various bipolar stimulators.

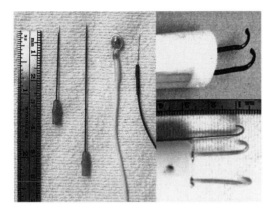

Fig. 5. Electrodes used to record CMAPs, NAPs, and SEPs.

current as 1 to 5 mA for a duration of 0.05 milliseconds. Overstimulation can produce excessive stimulus artifact, nonspecific stimulation of surrounding nerves, or stimulus spread along the course of the nerve. Diseased nerves typically have a higher threshold for stimulation. Orientation of the stimulator is also important. Bipolar stimulation produces a more focal distribution of current than monopolar stimulation and is therefore preferred for intraoperative stimulation of most peripheral nerves. The cathode and anode should be aligned with the long axis of the nerve, and the cathode should be proximal to the desired direction of the current.

Recording
CMAPs are recorded from surface, subcutaneous, or intramuscular needle electrodes (Fig. 5).

Intramuscular wire electrodes can also be used for selective recordings from deeper muscles.

Nerve action potentials (NAPs) are similar to SNAPs but record activity in both motor and sensory fibers directly from a mixed nerve. NAPs are recorded with a handheld bipolar recorder placed directly on the nerve, and SEPs are recorded from surface electrodes over the cervical spine and contralateral parietal scalp. CMAP recordings are large and less contaminated with artifact and exclusively monitor the function of motor axons (Fig. 6). NAPs reflect activity in motor and sensory axons, and SEPs record activity in sensory fibers. NAPs and SEPs are relatively small compared with CMAPs and often require averaging. NAP recordings pose a technical challenge because of excessive stimulus artifact, which is caused by the proximity of the stimulating and recording electrodes. At least 4 cm of separation is needed to record reliable NAPs intraoperatively. The following factors may reduce stimulus artifact: keeping stimulus intensities low, the use of a three-pronged electrode with a built-in ground, lifting the nerve away from moisture, and restricting the low- and high-frequency filters. The amplitude of the CMAP, NAP, and SEP responses are proportional to the number of functioning axons in their respective pathways. Table 1 summarizes the technical parameters used to record CMAPs, NAPs, and SEPs intraoperatively.

Motor evoked potentials
There are various techniques in use to record peripheral motor activity generated in central motor pathways. The most common stimulation methods involve transcranial electric or magnetic

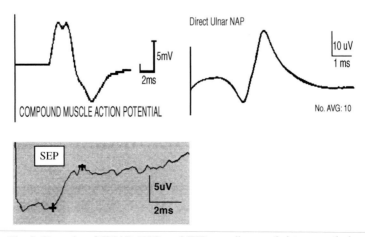

Fig. 6. Examples of CMAP, NAP, and SEP recordings made intraoperatively.

Table 1
Summary of intraoperative technical parameters

CMAPs, NAPs, SEPs	Stimulation	Recording
Electrodes	Direct stimulation with probe, hook, or plate electrodes: size and shape determined by nerve; bipolar configuration most common with cathode closest to recording electrode	CMAP: surface, subcutaneous, or intramuscular electrode NAP: subcutaneous or direct with probe, hook, or plate electrodes SEP: surface or subdermal needle electrodes over cervical spine and contralateral scalp (C3′ or C4′–Fz, C3′–C4′)
Parameters	Direct: 0.05 ms, 1–20 mA Frequency: single stimulus or 1.9–3.9 Hz	Filters: 30–1000 or 2000 Hz Average: 0–50 traces (NAP and SEP)
Technical problems	1. Stimulator failure, especially electrode orientation, location, and impedance; poor contact with nerve, excess fluid around site of stimulation 2. Overstimulation: stimulate wrong nerve 3. Stimulus artifact, obscures response 4. Peripheral ischemia (tourniquet), must wait minimum of 30 min after tourniquet released	1. Electrical noise: microscope, blood warmer, cautery, poor grounding 2. Electrode impedance too high, poor contact, excess fluid around recording electrode 3. Volume-conducted muscle response

Other factors

Effects of physiologic variables on CMAP or NAP	Age: none Anesthetics/drugs: neuromuscular blocking agents may obscure CMAPs, anesthetics may reduce scalp potential of SEP Blood pressure: none significant Temperature: increased latency of all responses but likely not significant for intraoperative diagnostic purposes
Pathophysiologic correlation	Root avulsion: presence of SEP with root stimulation indicates continuity of dorsal root and likely ventral root 1. Partial distal lesions: (1) CMAP/NAP/SEP size correlates with number of functioning axons; (2) increased latency or change in amplitude when stimulating "through" lesion, helpful in localization if distance and stimulus intensity tightly controlled; (3) stimulation/recording used to identify nerves when anatomy distorted and viable fascicles when feasible to spare them 2. Complete distal lesions: (1) CMAP/NAP/SEP absent in complete lesions without early regeneration, (2) NAP across injury site confirms early regeneration
Advantages	Adds significant localization and regeneration information to preoperative studies
Disadvantages	Technical problems may impair reliability; extra time required to perform reliable studies in surgical setting; requires patience of surgical team

stimulation of the cerebral cortex, although electrical stimulation of the spinal cord has been described and is currently the most widely used method to monitor spinal cord function during spine surgery. Until recently, transcranial stimulation was not approved for use in the United States without an investigative device exemption, but it has now been approved. Although recording has been traditionally from muscle, several groups have reported the recording of NAPs from various elements of the brachial plexus with transcranial electrical stimulation [5–7]. This technique has the theoretic advantage of determining the integrity of motor root function.

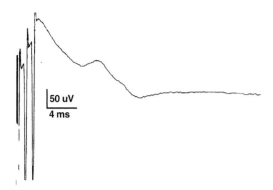

50 uV
4 ms

Fig. 7. Transcranial electrical MEPs recorded intra-operatively over the medial, lateral, and posterior cords of the brachial plexus. (*Adapted from* Burkholder LM, Houlden DA, Midha R, Weiss E, Vennettilli M. Neurogenic motor evoked potentials: role in brachial plexus surgery. J Neurosurg 2003;98:607–10; with permission.)

There are still technical hurdles to overcome before this technique can be applied routinely. One problem has been the exquisite sensitivity of MEPs to inhalation anesthetics. This problem can usually be solved by using narcotic-based anesthetic techniques, with limited use or total elimination of inhalation anesthetics. The most difficult problem with MEP recordings over the brachial plexus is excessive stimulus artifact, which

frequently obscures the NAP and requires recording over more distal elements rather than directly from the nerve roots [5]. Figure 7 shows an example of transcranial electrical MEPs recorded intraoperatively over the sixth cervical (C6) nerve root. In this patient with a severe plexopathy, there were motor NAPs recorded over the C6 root but none over the C5 or C7 roots. Nerve grafts therefore were placed between the C6 root to the axillary and musculocutaneous nerves.

Utility of electrophysiologic studies during brachial plexus surgery

Intraoperative studies using NCSs, SEPs, and possibly MEPs are particularly helpful during brachial plexus exploration and repair. Many of the limitations of preoperative electrodiagnostic studies outlined previously can be overcome with intraoperative studies.

Nerve root integrity

Most important, SEPs [8–10] and possibly MEPs [5–7] can be used to determine the presence or absence of nerve root avulsion. The repair of postganglionic elements in the setting of confirmed nerve root avulsion is of no benefit. A well-defined SEP recorded from the brain or spinal cord after direct stimulation of the exposed nerve root

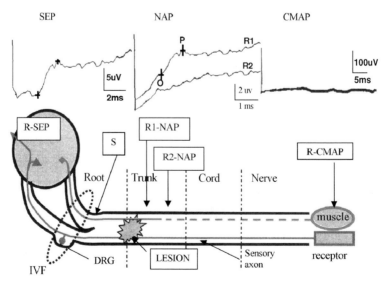

Fig. 8. Findings on SEP, NAP, and CMAP recordings in a partial axonal lesion affecting postganglionic elements of the brachial plexus. The nerve root is intact, and there is early regeneration through the lesion. The SEP documents that the root is intact. The presence of an NAP indicates axonal continuity through the lesion. The presence of a CMAP recorded over distal muscles indicates that the original lesion was incomplete. IVF, intervertebral foramen; R, record; S, stimulated.

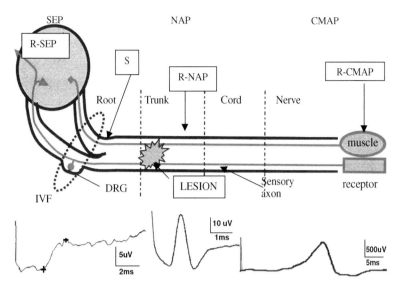

Fig. 9. Findings on SEP, NAP, and CMAP recordings in a complete axonal lesion affecting postganglionic elements of the brachial plexus. The nerve root is intact, and there is early regeneration through the lesion. The SEP documents that the root is intact. The presence of an NAP indicates early regeneration through the lesion. The absence of a CMAP recorded over distal muscles indicates that the original lesion was complete with no residual partial innervation. IVF, intervertebral foramen; R, record; S, stimulated.

indicates central continuity of the dorsal root [5,8–10]. In most cases, this finding indicates a high likelihood of ventral root continuity as well [5,10]. The recording of an NAP from plexus elements following transcranial electrical stimulation (MEP), however, provides more direct evidence of ventral root continuity (see Fig. 7) [5–7]. NAPs can also be used to assess root integrity indirectly [3,11], but the proper interpretation of an NAP in the setting of root avulsion requires experience and is not always definitive. The total absence of the NAP while stimulating the root and recording 4 cm distal along the spinal nerve or proximal trunk suggests root avulsion, but a very proximal postganglionic lesion could also produce this finding. Also, in root avulsion, if the postganglionic element is intact, a well-defined NAP will be recorded from preserved postganglionic sensory fibers. This recording is usually useful in differentiating a small, delayed NAP generated by early regeneration of axons across the site of injury, but inexperienced and unaware physicians could easily misinterpret these findings.

Assessment of partial and complete plexus lesions

Once nerve root continuity is confirmed, from a physiologic and prognostic point of view there are two main types of lesions that affect the more distal elements of the brachial plexus [3,11]. Partial lesions are incomplete and associated

with residual motor or sensory axonal continuity. Intraoperative NCS using CMAP or NAP recordings can help to determine the location and severity of partial lesions in brachial plexopathy. Using direct stimulation of plexus elements exposed at surgery, the fascicles of interest can be better isolated, allowing more precise segmental localization of partial lesions. In partial lesions, CMAPs, NAPs, and SEPs produce recordable responses across and distal to the injured segment (Fig. 8). The size of the response is proportional to the number of functioning axons. Most partial lesions are left alone or treated with external neurolysis. Complete lesions are associated with total axonal interruption at the time of injury. When brachial plexus surgery is performed several months post injury, complete lesions can be subdivided into those that show signs of regeneration across the injured segment and those that do not. NAP and SEP recordings are better suited

Table 2
Summary of intraoperative monitoring (IOM) studies: root lesions

Severity	CMAP	NAP	SEP	MEP[a]
Partial	±	+	+	+
Complete	−	−	−	−

Abbreviations: +, present; −, absent.
[a] Stimulating cortex, recording nerve.

Table 3
Summary of intraoperative monitoring (IOM) studies: lesions distal to root

Severity	CMAP	NAP	SEP	MEP[a]
Partial	+	+	+	+
Complete	−	+ If early regeneration − If no regeneration	+ If early regeneration − If no regeneration	+ If early regeneration − If no regeneration

Abbreviations: +, present; −, absent.
[a] Stimulating cortex, recording nerve.

than CMAP recordings in detecting early regeneration, because reinnervation at this stage typically has yet to reach a target muscle (Fig. 9). When regeneration is detected, the segment is left alone or external neurolysis is performed. If the NAP or SEP is absent, then grafting is performed, as long as proximal nerve root continuity is confirmed. The findings on various types of intraoperative recordings in partial and complete lesions are summarized in Tables 2 and 3.

In summary, electrodiagnostic studies performed preoperatively and during surgery complement one another and complement information provided by clinical and imaging studies in brachial plexus injury. The information provided by electrodiagnostic studies helps to better define the number, location, and severity of plexus lesions. In addition, establishing the presence or absence of nerve root continuity and early regeneration through postganglionic lesions is used to help direct surgical therapy.

References

[1] Brown WF, Veitch J. AAEM minimonograph 42: intraoperative monitoring of peripheral and cranial nerves. Muscle Nerve 1994;17:371–7.

[2] Daube JR, Harper CM. Surgical monitoring of cranial and peripheral nerves. In: Desmedt JE, editor. Neuromonitoring in surgery. Amsterdam: Elsevier; 1989. p. 115–51.

[3] Spinner RJ, Kline DG. Surgery for peripheral nerve and brachial plexus injuries or other nerve lesions. Muscle Nerve 2000;23:680–95.

[4] Tiel RL, Happel LT Jr, Kline DG. Nerve action potential recording method and equipment. Neurosurgery 1996;39:103–8.

[5] Burkholder LM, Houlden DA, Midha R, Weiss E, Vennettilli M. Neurogenic motor evoked potentials: role in brachial plexus surgery. J Neurosurg 2003;98:607–10.

[6] Turkof E, Monsivais J, Dechtyar I, Bellolo H, Millesi H, Mayr N. Motor evoked potential as a reliable method to verify the conductivity of anterior spinal roots in brachial plexus surgery: an experimental study on goats. J Reconstr Microsurg 1995;11:357–62.

[7] Turkof E, Millesi H, Turkof R. Intraoperative electroneurodiagnostics (transcranial electrical motor evoked potentials) to evaluate the functional status of anterior spinal roots and spinal nerves during brachial plexus surgery. Plast Reconstr Surg 1997;99:1632–41.

[8] Landi A, Copeland SA, Parry CB, Jones SJ. The role of somatosensory evoked potentials and nerve conduction studies in the surgical management of brachial plexus injuries. J Bone Joint Surg [Br] 1980;62:492–7.

[9] Sugioka H, Tsuyana N, Hara T, Nagano A, Tachibana S, Ochiai N. Investigation of brachial plexus injuries by intra-operative cortical somatosensory evoked potentials. Arch Orthop Trauma Surg 1982;99:143.

[10] Hashimoto T, Mitomo M, Hirabuki N, et al. Nerve root avulsion of birth palsy: comparison of myelography with CT myelography and somatosensory evoked potential. Radiology 1991;178:841–5.

[11] Kline DG. Surgical repair of peripheral nerve injury. Muscle Nerve 1990;13:843–52.

ELSEVIER
SAUNDERS

Hand Clin 21 (2005) 47–54

HAND
CLINICS

Planning Brachial Plexus Surgery: Treatment Options and Priorities

Robert H. Brophy, MD[a], Scott W. Wolfe, MD[a,b],*

[a]Hospital for Special Surgery, 535 East 70th Street, New York, NY 10021, USA
[b]Cornell-Weill Medical Center, 525 East 68th Street, New York, NY 10021, USA

Brachial plexus injuries are devastating and strike a predominantly young, active population. These injuries are most often caused by high-energy motorcycle and motor vehicle accidents. Although such injuries have plagued mankind for centuries, as evidenced by their description in the *Iliad*, little progress had been made in their management and treatment until the last few decades. Advances in basic science and anatomy during and following World War II set the stage for breakthrough progress in surgical techniques starting in the 1960s. This progress has led to increasingly successful clinical intervention for these otherwise catastrophic injuries. A crucial aspect of improving outcomes has been careful preparation for surgery, including accurate classification of the injury, appropriate timing of the intervention, and precise preoperative planning.

Injury classification

Brachial plexus injuries can be divided into two broad categories: supraclavicular injuries and infraclavicular injuries (Fig. 1). Supraclavicular injuries are more common and represent 70% to 75% of traumatic brachial plexus injuries. These injuries result most often from a traction mechanism, and patients are unlikely to recover without surgery. Half of supraclavicular injuries involve all five spinal levels (C5–T1) [1]. Of these complete five-level injuries, most (60%) are upper trunk (C5–C6/7) rupture in combination with lower

trunk (C7/8–T1) avulsion. Approximately 30% of these injuries are true complete five-level avulsion injuries, and the remaining 10% are actually C4 through T1 complete avulsion injuries with a very poor prognosis.

The most common pattern of incomplete supraclavicular injury is an upper trunk palsy. These types of injuries represent approximately 35% of all supraclavicular injuries and are typically characterized by avulsion or proximal rupture of C5/C6, with or without an injury of C7. The lower trunk is characteristically spared, or recovers relatively quickly from a transient neuropraxia. The avulsion of C6-C8, with sparing or recovery of C5 and T1, occurs much less frequently and represents 8% of all supraclavicular injuries. Isolated C8 and T1 avulsion or trunk rupture is rare, occurring in only 3% of all supraclavicular injuries. It is important to remember that 15% of supraclavicular injuries have concomitant segmental injuries at or below the clavicle where the peripheral nerves branch from the plexus [2]. The musculocutaneous, axillary, and suprascapular nerves are particularly vulnerable to traction injury because of soft tissue tethers near their origins. In addition, a prefixed (C4 contribution to the upper trunk) or postfixed (T2 contribution to the lower trunk) plexus may confuse the presentation of a supraclavicular injury.

Infraclavicular injuries constitute 25% to 33% of brachial plexus injuries [1–3]. These injuries tend to occur at the level of the cords or peripheral nerves and are usually incomplete. They are often caused by shoulder fractures or dislocations. Almost half (45%) are considered whole limb injuries and are frequently associated with shoulder trauma, including fracture-dislocation,

* Corresponding author. Hospital for Special Surgery, 535 East 70th Street, New York, NY 10021.
E-mail address: wolfes@hss.edu (S.W. Wolfe).

0749-0712/05/$ - see front matter © 2005 Elsevier Inc. All rights reserved.
doi:10.1016/j.hcl.2004.09.007

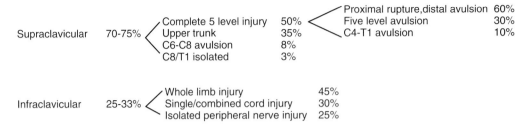

Fig. 1. Distribution of location and type of brachial plexus injuries.

scapulothoracic dissociation, or clavicular fractures. Approximately 30% are single or combined cord injuries. Isolated peripheral nerve palsies of the axillary, radial, or musculocutaneous nerve make up the remaining 25% of infraclavicular injuries. It is important to remember that 5% to 25% of infraclavicular injuries are associated with concomitant rupture or thrombosis of the axillary artery [1–3].

Brachial plexus injuries caused by penetrating trauma usually occur in the infraclavicular plexus, although any combination of injury to different levels of the plexus can be seen. Gunshot wounds (GSWs) usually cause neuropraxic injury to the plexus. Iatrogenic injuries can be seen related to various procedures. For example, resection of the first rib can be associated with injury at the division or cord level. Axillary lymph node dissection may endanger the long thoracic or thoracodorsal nerves, and cervical lymph node biopsy is frequently complicated by injury to the spinal accessory nerve. Shoulder procedures, especially stabilization or capsular release, may occasionally be associated with injuries of the axillary, median, or radial nerves.

Spontaneous recovery within 1 year is more likely in infraclavicular injuries than in supraclavicular injuries. It has been suggested that these injuries are more likely to recover because they occur farther from the nerve's "anchorage" point [3], and are thus less likely to involve nerve disruption. Surgery is generally not necessary in closed cord injuries below the clavicle. It is important to remember, however, that the axillary nerve is tethered at the quadrangular space and thus more vulnerable to axonal injury. Isolated axillary nerve injuries have a less favorable recovery rate and may require surgical intervention, including exploration and possibly excision and grafting. Similarly, the musculocutaneous nerve is tethered where it enters the coracobrachialis, and the suprascapular nerve is tethered at the suprascapular notch.

Timing of surgical intervention

Perhaps the most crucial aspect of planning surgical intervention for brachial plexus injury is selecting the timing of surgery.

Indications for acute exploration include the following: concomitant vascular injury, open injuries caused by sharp laceration, and crush or contaminated open wounds. With crush or contaminated wounds, it is advisable to identify and tag divided nerve stumps for later repair. Devitalized tissue should be debrided and bony injuries stabilized, and any accompanying arterial injuries should be repaired primarily. Early exploration, within 1 to 2 weeks, is recommended for unequivocal, complete C5-T1 avulsion injuries [4]. Plexus injuries that occur from a low-energy GSW are generally neuropraxic and should not be routinely explored.

Delayed exploration (3 mo after the initial injury) is recommended for complete injuries with no recovery by clinical examination or electromyography (EMG) at 12 weeks post injury. Other candidates for exploration are those who show distal recovery without regaining clinical or electrical evidence of proximal muscle function. Patients with iatrogenic injury, as may occur following neck exploration or lymph node biopsy, should also be explored relatively early, particularly if electrodiagnostic testing shows complete denervation without evidence of recovering motor unit potentials.

Nerve reconstruction is not routinely recommended in adults more than 9 months after the inciting injury [5–10], although reconstruction has been attempted in patients up to 12 months later [11], and some authors have reported results of patients treated more than 12 months after their initial trauma [9,12,13]. One study found a statistically significant difference in the average time from injury to surgery between patients with successful outcomes, treated, on average, 4.3 months after their initial accident, when compared with patients with unsuccessful outcomes, treated at an average of 6.3 months after injury ($P = 0.003$) [5]. Another study showed significantly better biceps strength in patients treated within 6 months of their injury compared with patients treated more than 12 months after their injury ($P < 0.05$) [9].

Age is an important variable to consider with regards to timing of brachial plexus surgery. Some authors have suggested that an age of more than 50 years is a contraindication for surgical exploration [13]. Other authors have reported encouraging results with older patients [11,12]. One study, which reported on 63 patients with a mean age of 23 years and an age range of 10 to 52 years, found no statistically significant relationship between clinical outcome and the age of the patient [5]. As a general rule, most surgeons are more likely to operate on younger patients, and younger patients tend to do better than older patients. Thus, younger patients tend to be offered more aggressive surgical options even later after the initial injury than older patients.

Preoperative planning

Physical examination

Once the decision has been made to operate, careful preoperative planning with the entire surgical team is essential (Box 1). Clinical records should be examined with special attention to the patient's postinjury physical examination and subsequent recovery, if any. Careful and repeated evaluation of upper extremity motor and sensory function is mandatory.

When evaluating supraclavicular lesions, it is important to differentiate between avulsion and extraforaminal injuries. Although abrasions and

---

Box 1. Preoperative planning priorities for brachial plexus injury surgery

1. Review clinical examinations
2. Scrutinize electrodiagnostic studies
3. Review CT myelography/imaging
4. Assemble operative team, plan for intraoperative electrodiagnostic studies
5. Plan a preoperative conference, including priorities and contingency plans
6. Prepare patient's expectations

---

ecchymosis in the posterior triangle of the neck are commonly seen in both types of injury, a positive Tinel's sign suggests extraforaminal injury. Root avulsion or preganglionic injury is suggested by numerous findings, including an elevated hemidiaphragm and lost sensation above the clavicle. Horner's syndrome suggests an avulsion injury to the lower two roots. Fractures of the C7 transverse process or the first rib are also associated with preganglionic injury to the lower two roots. The head may tilt away from the injured side, which indicates complete five-level intradural injury. The presence of unremitting deafferentation pain, described by patients as burning or crushing in character, also supports a diagnosis of preganglionic injury. Paradoxically, peripheral sympathetic tone may be preserved, because the sympathetic cell bodies reside in the sympathetic trunk, outside of the cord and distal to the zone of injury.

Different physical examination findings are associated with infraclavicular injuries. There may be sparing of peripheral nerves originating from the cords—for example, the subscapularis nerves (upper, middle, lower) and the pectoral nerves (medial, lateral). Patients may have decreased or absent peripheral sympathetic tone. A strongly positive Tinel's sign is almost always present in an infraclavicular lesion.

Electrodiagnostic studies

Electrodiagnostic studies should be reviewed in detail to document the level and extent of injury. Somatosensory evoked potentials (SEPs) and sensory nerve action potentials have been used to help determine the location of brachial plexus lesions [14,15]. EMG can be used to assess the peripheral and paraspinal musculature. Denervated rhomboids, serratus anterior, and trapezius all suggest avulsion of the C5-7 roots. A repeat EMG at least 6 weeks after an initial EMG is helpful to look for spontaneous recovery. Intact proximal musculature or recovery in proximal musculature suggests intact rootlets, as does the presence of at least some distal motor function. Sensory nerve conduction studies can be helpful, because preserved sensory conduction in the presence of anesthesia strongly supports a preganglionic supraclavicular injury.

Imaging studies

All imaging studies should be reviewed, with an emphasis on differentiating between pre- and postganglionic injuries. Myelography, CT myelography, and MRI are particularly helpful for this purpose. No imaging modality has been shown to be clearly superior, especially if used alone, although given a choice of only one modality, most brachial plexus surgeons would probably select CT myelography (Fig. 2). Nagano et al [16] showed an association between progressive myelographic abnormalities and preganglionic injury, with 90% of normal-appearing roots found to be postganglionic injury, whereas a traumatic meningocele was associated with preganglionic injury 98% of the time. Intermediate findings were associated with lesser rates of accuracy. CT myelography has been shown to have accuracy ranging from 70% to 95% [12,17–20]. Assessing the C8 and T1 roots is more difficult with CT myelography, because of the increasing obliquity of the more caudal spinal nerves and signal artifact arising in short, stout necks [21]. Using myelography in combination with CT myelography is likely to be more accurate. MRI is considered less accurate than CT myelography for detecting nerve root avulsion [12,21,22], although MRI is noninvasive and visualizes the extraforaminal plexus [23]. Hems et al [24] reported that a normal MRI of the supraclavicular plexus excludes significant postganglionic injury. Research continues into improving techniques for MRI imaging of brachial plexus lesions [21,25].

Logistics and prioritization

While reviewing the diagnostic data, the operative team needs to be organized, including making arrangements for intraoperative

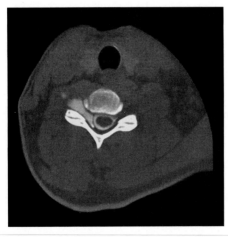

Fig. 2. CT myelogram of nerve root avulsion.

electrodiagnostic testing. A preoperative conference is helpful for assigning intraoperative priorities, developing an operative plan, and preparing contingency plans for possible intraoperative complications.

Prioritization is essential. First, it is important to clearly understand the anatomy of the injured plexus in each patient. It is equally important to identify what is available for possible nerve transfer. The surgeon must ask what is realistic to expect for a given patient, because it is important to set the patient's goals for any operation in line with the surgical expectations.

For functional priorities, it is generally agreed that elbow flexion is the most important function to restore. Active shoulder control is considered next most important, with abduction, external rotation, and scapular stabilization prioritized in that order. Long thoracic nerve reinnervation should be performed whenever possible. Proximal radial nerve motor function can often be restored, with triceps function more likely to return than wrist and finger extension. Restoring useful ulnar and median nerve motor function is not a consistently realistic goal for surgical intervention, although experimental efforts are focusing on this area. Sensation in the median nerve distribution should be restored if at all possible, and this factor has been shown to relieve pain in multilevel avulsion injuries, even in the absence of functional median nerve motor recovery. Berman et al [26] described late (>1 y post injury) intercostal nerve transfer for the sole purpose of pain relief in patients with brachial plexus injury. Significant relief was noted in 16 of 19 patients an average of 8 months after transfer.

Surgical options

Once the priorities for returning function have been assigned, the options for restoring function need to be explored. The authors focus on surgical options for restoring the function of the brachial plexus, including neurolysis, nerve repair, nerve grafting, and nerve transfer.

Neurolysis can be done, but it is rarely able to restore function as an isolated intervention. Narakas [27] found that neurolysis was effective only if scar tissue was observed around the nerve or inside the epineurium, preventing recovery or causing pain. Pre- and postneurolysis direct nerve stimulation is mandatory to evaluate improvement in nerve conduction. Clinically, it is often difficult to assess the efficacy of neurolysis because improvement may also be from spontaneous recovery.

Nerve repair is not a viable option in most subacute or delayed cases and should be considered only in sharp transections with excellent fascicular pattern and minimal scar. Tension on the repair is detrimental to recovery and should be avoided.

Nerve graft is indicated for well-defined ruptured nerve ends without segmental injury. Intraoperatively, a good fascicular pattern should be seen after the neuroma is excised. A portion of the resected nerve can be sent to pathology for intraoperative evaluation of the degree of scarring and the viability of the remaining fascicles. SEPs should show conductivity of stimulated roots [14,15,28,29]. Possible sources for nerve graft include the sural, antebrachial cutaneous, radial sensory, and possibly the ulnar nerve. The sural nerve can provide up to 40 cm of cable material. The donor nerve should be left in situ until the recipient bed is prepared. Before implantation, the graft orientation should be reversed to minimize axonal branch loss. Generally, shorter grafts (<10 cm) result in more successful outcomes than longer grafts [5,9,30,31], although one study found no relationship between graft length (≤25 cm) and graft success [32] when restoring function to the deltoid and biceps. Nerve grafting for distal function has been less successful compared with grafts to restore proximal function [32]. Vascularized nerve grafts have not been shown to achieve superior results compared with free-nerve grafts [33]. Surgical technique is considered the most important factor influencing results of nerve grafts [9], with the goal of perfect coaptation with no tension at the nerve union site.

Nerve transfer, or neurotization, options include intraplexal and extraplexal sources. Plexoplexal options include the undamaged roots, which often have to be confirmed intraoperatively with electrodiagnostic testing. Other options include the medial pectoral nerve and medial cord/ulnar nerve. Oberlin et al [34] described the anastomosis of one or two fascicles of the ulnar nerve to the biceps. Extraplexal options include the spinal accessory nerve and intercostal nerves. The phrenic nerve is also an option, and the motor branches of the deep cervical plexus (C3-4) can be used as donors as well. With the exception of the deep cervical plexus, all of these options have been shown in one or more reports to restore M3 or better elbow flexion in nearly two thirds of patients [11–13].

A plan to use undamaged roots requires contingency planning in the event of unexpected findings on intraoperative electrodiagnostic studies. The Oberlin technique is indicated for patients with upper trunk avulsion and no lower trunk injury [13], and the use of one or two fascicles of the ulnar nerve has not been reported to show a significant motor or sensory deficit postoperatively [34–36]. Success rates reported with the Oberlin transfer have been very good, with 94% to 100% of patients achieving M3 or better biceps strength, and 75% to 94% achieving at least M4 biceps strength [34–36]. The procedure requires an intact lower plexus, however. As an alternative, the spinal accessory nerve is a pure motor nerve, but its use is limited to one or two of its distal branches so as to preserve important upper trapezius function. On occasion, high-energy injuries may be associated with disruption of the spinal accessory nerve; this situation is usually evidenced by severe atrophy on physical examination. There is no known deficit associated with intercostal nerve transfer, but these small nerves may be damaged in patients with pneumothorax, chest tube, multiple rib fractures, or concomitant spinal cord injury. The phrenic nerve is attractive as a donor because it is a pure motor nerve with abundant axons, but its use carries the theoretic risk of endangering respiratory function, especially in patients who undergo simultaneous intercostal nerve transfer. A study by Gu et al [37] showed no measurable decrement in pulmonary function after phrenic nerve transfer. Transferring the motor branches of the C3-4 cervical plexus may endanger any remaining scapular stability in patients with five-level avulsion injuries.

Contralateral C7 transfer is another option, and preliminary results have been encouraging [38–40]. The clinical indication is a complete plexopathy with multiple avulsions and limited donor possibilities. The contralateral C7 root can be extended by means of a vascularized ulnar nerve graft in patients with C8-T1 avulsions, and the median nerve is the most frequent recipient. Donor deficits have been reported, including biceps and triceps motor and C7 sensory function, although the risk is currently not considered significant [39,41,42].

Another option is transferring the nerve to the long head of the triceps to the anterior branch of the axillary nerve to restore deltoid motor function, as described by Witoonchart et al [43] and Leechavengvongs et al [44]. This transfer has been shown to be anatomically feasible [43] and clinically promising when used in conjunction with spinal accessory nerve transfer to the suprascapular nerve [44].

Once the potential nerve transfer donors have been identified, the surgeon must match these with realistic targets for reinnervation. The spinal accessory nerve can be repaired to the suprascapular nerve or to the musculocutaneous nerve. The phrenic nerve or an undamaged C5 root can be used to reinnervate the axillary nerve. Intercostals can be used for various combinations of the musculocutaneous, long thoracic, radial, or median nerves. Contralateral C7 transfer is usually for the median nerve. The nerve to the long head of the triceps is transferred to the anterior branch of the axillary nerve.

One important factor for these nerve transfers is the number of axons available in possible donors [45]. The number of myelinated nerve axons in a single branch to the pectoral muscle is roughly 400 to 600, whereas the phrenic nerve contains 800 of these axons. One intercostal nerve contains 1300 myelinated axons, the long thoracic nerve 1600, and the spinal accessory nerve 1700 myelinated axons. The motor branches of the deep cervical plexus contain 3400 to 4000 myelinated axons, and C7 may hold between 16,000 and 40,000 mixed motor and sensory axons. The nerve to the long head of the triceps contains an average of roughly 1200 axon fibers [43]. In comparison, a typical recipient, such as the musculocutaneous nerve, is composed of approximately 6000 motor axons [9]. The anterior branch of the axillary nerve has been shown to contain an average of 2700 axons [43].

Patient expectations

Managing patient expectations is perhaps the most important part of preoperative planning and preparation. Patients need to understand the limits of the best possible outcome and the possibility that no or limited functional improvement may occur after surgery. Prognosis is highly dependent on the pattern of injury. Complete C4 to T1 injuries are considered the most severe and are virtually irreparable, but these injuries are uncommon. Avulsion injuries from C5 to T1 have been shown to be amenable to restoration of shoulder and elbow function, but distal function is virtually impossible to restore with current techniques. Proximal root rupture with distal root avulsion also allows for recovery of shoulder and elbow function, and patients may recover some

sensation and get relief of pain. The ideal candidates for surgery are patients with proximal rupture or avulsion and sparing of the lower trunk. These patients retain hand function and often get good shoulder and elbow function. Infraclavicular lesions are amenable to direct repair and may require nerve grafting for segmental defects. Nerve transfers are usually not necessary.

Summary

Brachial plexus injuries are devastating and usually result from high-energy trauma in young patients. Clinicians treating brachial plexus injuries need to recognize the pattern of injury presenting in each patient. Most injuries can be described as either supraclavicular or infraclavicular. The specific injury is determined by means of a precise workup, including careful physical examination, electrodiagnostic studies, and imaging studies; a thorough workup is essential for successful preoperative planning. Priorities need to be identified and matched with available resources in each patient. A growing number of good treatment alternatives are available. Finally, counseling patients toward realistic expectations is a critical component of preparation for surgery.

References

[1] Birch R. Brachial plexus injuries. J Bone Joint Surg Br 1995;78(6):986–92.

[2] Alnot JY. Traumatic brachial plexus palsy in the adult: retro- and infraclavicular lesions. Clin Orthop 1988;237:9–16.

[3] Leffert RD, Seddon H. Infraclavicular brachial plexus injuries. J Bone Joint Surg Br 1965;47(1): 9–22.

[4] Megalon G, Bordeaux J, Legre R, Aubert JP. Emergency versus delayed repair of severe brachial plexus injuries. Clin Orthop 1988;237:32–5.

[5] Bentolila V, Nizard R, Bizot P, Sedel L. Complete traumatic brachial plexus palsy. Treatment and outcome after repair. J Bone Joint Surg Am 1999;81(1): 20–8.

[6] Millesi H. Brachial plexus injuries. Nerve grafting. Clin Orthop 1988;237:36–42.

[7] Millesi H. Interfascicular grafts for repair of peripheral nerves of the upper extremity. Orthop Clin North Am 1977;8(2):387–404.

[8] Nagano A, Tsuyama N, Ochiai N, Hara T, Takahashi M. Direct nerve crossing with the intercostal nerve to treat avulsion injuries of the brachial plexus. J Hand Surg Am 1989;14(6):980–5.

[9] Samii M, Carvalho GA, Nikkhah G, Penkert G. Surgical reconstruction of the musculocutaneous

nerve in traumatic brachial plexus injuries. J Neurosurg 1997;87(6):881–6.

[10] Songcharoen P, Mahaisavariya T, Chotigavanich C. Spinal accessory neurotization for restoration of elbow flexion in avulsion injuries of the brachial plexus. J Hand Surg Am 1996;21(3):387–90.

[11] Merrell GA, Barrie KA, Katz DL, Wolfe SW. Results of nerve transfer techniques for restoration of shoulder and elbow function in the context of a meta-analysis of the English literature. J Hand Surg Am 2001;26(2):303–14.

[12] Dubuisson AS, Kline DG. Brachial plexus injury: a survey of 100 consecutive cases from a single service. Neurosurgery 2002;51(3):673–83.

[13] Nagano A. Treatment of brachial plexus injury. J Orthop Sci 1998;3(1):71–80.

[14] Jones SJ, Parry CB, Landi A. Diagnosis of brachial plexus traction lesions by sensory nerve action potentials and somatosensory evoked potentials. Injury 1981;12(5):376–82.

[15] Synek VM, Cowan JC. Somatosensory evoked potentials in patients with supraclavicular brachial plexus injuries. Neurology 1982;32(12):1347–52.

[16] Nagano A, Ochiai N, Sugioka H, Hara T. Usefulness of myelography in brachial plexus injuries. J Hand Surg Br 1989;14:59–64.

[17] Carvalho GA, Nikkhah G, Matthies G, Penkert G, Samii M. Diagnosis of root avulsions in traumatic brachial plexus injuries: value of computerized tomography myelography and magnetic resonance imaging. J Neurosurg 1997;86(1):69–76.

[18] Marshall RW, De Silva RDD. Computerised axial tomography in traction injuries of the brachial plexus. J Bone Joint Surg Br 1986;68(5):734–8.

[19] Oberle J, Antoniadis G, Rath SA, et al. Radiological investigations and intra-operative evoked potentials for the diagnosis of nerve root avulsion: evaluation of both modalities by intradural root inspection. Acta Neurochir 1998;140(6):527–31.

[20] Walker AT, Chaloupka JC, de De Lotbiniere ACJ, Wolfe SW, Goldman R, Kier EL. Detection of nerve rootlet avulsion on CT myelography in patients with birth palsy and brachial plexus injury after trauma. AJR Am J Roentgenol 1996;167(5):1283–7.

[21] Tavakkolizadeh A, Saifuddin A, Birch R. Imaging of adult brachial plexus traction injuries. J Hand Surg Br 2001;26(3):183–91.

[22] van Es HW. MRI of the brachial plexus. Eur Radiol 2001;11(2):325–36.

[23] Gupta RK, Mehta VS, Banerji AK, Jain RK. MR evaluation of brachial plexus injuries. Neuroradiology 1989;31(5):377–81.

[24] Hems TE, Birch R, Carlstedt T. The role of MRI in the management of traction injuries of the adult brachial plexus. J Hand Surg Br 1999;24(5):550–5.

[25] Doi K, Otsuka K, Okamoto Y, Fujii H, Hattori Y, Baliarsing AS. Cervical root avulsion in brachial plexus injuries: magnetic resonance imaging classification and comparison with myelography and computerized tomography myelography. J Neurosurg 2002;96(3 Suppl):277–84.

[26] Berman J, Anand P, Chen L, Taggart M, Birch R. Pain relief from preganglionic injury to the brachial plexus by late intercostal nerve transfer. J Bone Joint Surg Br 1996;78(5):759–60.

[27] Narakas A. Brachial plexus surgery. Orthop Clin North Am 1981;12(2):303–23.

[28] Turkof E, Millesi H, Turkof R, Pfundner P, Mayr N. Intraoperative electrodiagnostics (transcranial electrical motor evoked potentials) to evaluate the functional status of anterior spinal roots and spinal nerves during brachial plexus surgery. Plast Reconstr Surg 1997;99(6):1632–41.

[29] Turkof E, Monsivais J, Dechtyar I, Bellolo H, Millesi H, Mayr N. Motor evoked potential as a reliable method to verify the conductivity of anterior spinal roots in brachial plexus surgery: an experimental study on goats. J Reconstr Microsurg 1995;11(5):357–62.

[30] Chuang DC, Epstein MD, Yeh MC, Wei FC. Functional restoration of elbow flexion in brachial plexus injuries: results in 167 patients (excluding obstetric brachial plexus injury). J Hand Surg Am 1993; 18(2):285–91.

[31] Hentz VR, Narakas A. The results of microneurosurgical reconstruction in complete brachial plexus palsy: assessing outcome and predicting results. Orthop Clin North Am 1988;19(1):107–14.

[32] Ochiai N, Nagano A, Sugioka H, Hara T. Nerve grafting in brachial plexus injuries. Results of free grafts in 90 patients. J Bone Joint Surg Br 1996; 78(5):754–8.

[33] Birch R, Dunkerton M, Bonney G, Jamieson AM. Experience with the free vascularised ulnar nerve graft in repair of supraclavicular lesions of the brachial plexus. Clin Orthop 1988;237:96–104.

[34] Oberlin C, Beal D, Leechavengvongs S, Salon A, Dauge MC, Sarcy JJ. Nerve transfer to biceps muscle using a part of ulnar nerve for C5-C6 avulsion of the brachial plexus: anatomical study and report of four cases. J Hand Surg Am 1994; 19(2):232–7.

[35] Leechavengvongs S, Witoonchart K, Uerpairojkit C, Thuvasethakul P, Ketmalasiri W. Nerve transfer to biceps muscle using a part of the ulnar nerve in brachial plexus injury (upper arm type): a report of 32 cases. J Hand Surg Am 1998; 23(4):711–6.

[36] Sungpet A, Suphachatwong C, Kawinwonggowit V, Patradul A. Transfer of a single fascicle from the ulnar nerve to the biceps muscle after avulsions of upper roots of the brachial plexus. J Hand Surg Br 2000;25(4):325–8.

[37] Gu YD, Wu MM, Zhen YL, et al. Phrenic nerve transfer for brachial plexus motor neurotization. Microsurgery 1989;10(4):287–9.

[38] Gu Y, Xu J, Chen L, Wang H, Hu S. Long term outcome of contralateral C7 transfer: a report of 32 cases. Chin Med J 2002;115(6):866–8.

[39] Songcharoen P, Wongtrakul S, Mahaisavariya B, Spinner RJ. Hemicontralateral C7 transfer to median nerve in the treatment of root avulsion brachial plexus injury. J Hand Surg Am 2001;26(6):1058–64.

[40] Waikakul S, Orapin A, Vanadurongwan V. Clinical results of contralateral C7 root neurotization to the median nerve in brachial plexus injuries with total root avulsions. J Hand Surg Br 1999;24(5):556–60.

[41] Chuang DC, Cheng SL, Wei FC, Wu CL, Ho YS. Clinical evaluation of C7 spinal nerve transection: 21 patients with at least 2 years' follow-up. Br J Plast Surg 1998;51(4):285–90.

[42] Gu YD, Chen DS, Zhang GM, et al. Long-term functional results of contralateral C7 transfer. J Reconstr Microsurg 1998;14(1):57–9.

[43] Witoonchart K, Leechavengvongs S, Uerpairojkit C, Thuvasethakul P, Wongnopsuwan V. Nerve transfer to deltoid muscle using the nerve to the long head of the triceps, part I: an anatomic feasibility study. J Hand Surg Am 2003;28(4):628–32.

[44] Leechavengvongs S, Witoonchart K, Uerpairojkit C, Thuvasethakul P. Nerve transfer to deltoid muscle using the nerve to the long head of the triceps, part II: a report of 7 cases. J Hand Surg Am 2003; 28(4):633–8.

[45] Chuang DC. Neurotization procedures for brachial plexus injuries. Hand Clin 1995;11(4):633–45.

ELSEVIER
SAUNDERS

Hand Clin 21 (2005) 55–69

Direct Plexus Repair by Grafts Supplemented by Nerve Transfers

David G. Kline, MD[a,b,c,d],*, Robert L. Tiel, MD[a,b,c,d]

[a]Department of Neurosurgery, Louisiana State University Health Sciences Center, 1542 Tulane Avenue,
Box T7-3, New Orleans, LA 70112-2822, USA
[b]MCLNO Hospital, 1532 Tulane Avenue, New Orleans, LA 70112, USA
[c]Ochsner Hospital, 1516 Jefferson Highway, New Orleans, LA 70121, USA
[d]Touro Hospital, 1401 Foucher Street, New Orleans, LA 70115, USA

There is much literature available concerning nerve transfers for plexus stretch injures, which recently has been thoroughly analyzed [1]. Nonetheless, when injury to the plexus requiring repair is caused more by focal damage, such as laceration or gunshot wound (GSW), direct repair either with or without grafts is usually preferable to substitution for loss by nerve transfers. Thus, in many cases where one or more plexus elements were transected or in a relatively large panel of brachial plexus injuries caused by GSWs, and where elements were still in continuity but did not conduct a nerve action potential (NAP), direct repair, usually by grafts, has been the current authors' standard [2,3]. This approach also has been used in the past for stretch injuries before the use of nerve transfers was popularized [4–8]. Thus, an accounting of the reasoning and outcomes for direct repair is important, even for today's clinicians dealing with stretch or avulsion injury to the plexus. Finally, this article describes the approach used by the authors in recent years for stretch injuries, which involves direct repair of plexus elements, whenever possible supplemented by nerve transfers.

Methods

During a 30-year period (1968–1998) at Louisiana State University Health Sciences Center (LSUHSC), 1019 adult patients with plexus injury,

tumors, or presumed entrapment underwent surgery (Table 1). Although one half of these patients (509) had stretch or contusion as their mechanism of injury, 12% had GSWs involving the plexus (118 patients), and 7% (71 patients) had plexus laceration. The remainder, or 321, operative patients were equally divided by mechanism between tumor (161 patients) and thoracic outlet (160 patients). Thirty patients had iatrogenic injury involving either transection or contusion/stretch and avulsion and were incorporated under either plexus laceration or stretch/contusion categories. Excluded from this analysis were birth palsies because the management of these patients differs in some respects from adults with stretch injuries. Some of the following analysis was recently published and is redistilled for this article [9].

In addition to clinical workup and electromyographic (EMG) studies for each category of injury, stretch/contusion injuries were evaluated by myelography followed by CT scan cuts. There is a false-positive and false-negative incidence of findings, even with CT myelography, but these studies usually provided reliable information about each plexus root and whether avulsion or injury close to the spinal cord was likely. EMG studies were done in each patient 2 to 4 weeks post injury and included paraspinal and extremity muscle sampling and sensory conduction studies but seldom included noninvasive somatosensory studies [10].

At the time of surgery for supraclavicular stretch injuries, the current authors dissect out the elements in a 360° fashion and make direct recordings by stimulating proximal spinal nerve and recording from distal trunks or divisions and

* Corresponding author. Department of Neurosurgery, Louisiana State University Health Sciences Center, 1542 Tulane Avenue, Box T7-3, New Orleans, LA 70112-2822.

E-mail address: dkline@lsuhsc.edu (D.G. Kline).

Table 1
Operated brachial plexus lesions[a]

Type of lesion	No. of patients
Stretch/contusion	509 (50%)
Supraclavicular	366
Infraclavicular	143
Gunshot wound	118 (12%)
Laceration	71 (7%)
Thoracic outlet syndrome	160 (16%)
Tumor	161 (16%)
Total	1019 (100%)

Percentages indicated in parentheses indicate percentage of total number.
[a] LSUHSC series 1968–1998.

cords. If the trace is flat, then injury is either postganglionic or pre- and postganglionic, and the authors section proximal spinal nerve looking for usable fascicular structure for lead-out to grafts, which are usually harvested by using sural nerves. If the NAPs are positive but small in amplitude and slow in conduction, the element is regenerating and is not sectioned. If the response has high amplitude and is rapid in conduction, preganglionic injury with sensory fiber sparing is likely unless there has been preoperative clinical or EMG evidence of sparing in its distribution. This finding suggests that it is an intact or partially injured element. When NAP recordings are positive, the element (usually spinal nerve) is not sectioned in looking for fascicular structure unless visual inspection suggests the possibility of split repair, which is unusual in the stretch/contusion category. In the authors' experience, repairs were usually done with an interfasicular technique and donor nerves were usually sural, although, if healthy, the antebrachial cutaneous nerves were sometimes used [11].

Approximately 93% of patients returned for postoperative follow-up at least once. Subsequent visits were made by 70% of these patients, whereas others had a secondary follow-up by telephone in 20% and mail in 10% of cases. The minimal follow-up period was 18 months but averaged 4.2 years. Most of these follow-ups were in-person evaluations performed by the senior author, but some follow-up after 3 years post surgery was performed by other physicians closer to the patient's home or, in a few instances, by phone or mail with the patient or his or her family.

Results

The LSUHSC system for evaluating outcomes in plexus lesions was used (Box 1). This system

---

Box 1. System of grading by elements of brachial plexus

0: no muscle contraction
1 (poor): proximal muscles contract but not against gravity
2 (fair): proximal muscles contract against gravity, distal muscles do not contract; sensory grade, if applicable, was usually 2 or lower
3 (moderate): proximal muscles contract against gravity and some resistance; some distal muscles contract against gravity; sensory grade, if applicable, was usually 3
4 (good): all muscles contract against gravity and some resistance; sensory grade, if applicable, was 3 or 4
5 (excellent): all muscles contract against moderate resistance; sensory grade, if applicable, was 4 or better

---

differs from the Medical Research Council (MRC) system in that LSUHSC grade 3 includes at least some muscle contraction against mild resistance and gravity, whereas a grade 2 is against gravity only, which would correspond to an MRC grade 3. Favorable outcomes were therefore determined in patients with elements recovering to an LSUHSC grade of 3 or better level not to an MRC grade 3.

Lacerations

Outcomes in which the mechanism was from presumed laceration by glass, knife, or other sharp object (sharp) versus propeller blades, chain saws, or auto metal (blunt) are seen in Table 2. Data combine unfavorable with favorable elements for repair by suture versus grafts, or neurolysis based on NAPs across contused but not lacerated elements. Thus, outcomes with lower plexus elements, such as C8, T1 spinal nerves and medial cord, were blended with those with more favorable elements for repair.

Table 2 shows reasonably favorable outcomes for suture: 81% of elements recovered to a grade 3 or better level if the laceration was sharp and the repair was done within 72 hours, and 70% of elements recovered to this level after delayed or secondary end-to-end suture. Delayed repair by grafts had grade 3 or better outcomes in 53% of elements. If sharp transection could be explored

Table 2
Surgical outcome in brachial plexus lacerations[a]

	Elements in continuity	Sharp transection	Blunt transection	Totals
Plexus cases	20	28	23	71
Plexus elements	57	83	61	201
Neurolysis (+NAPs)	24/26	0/0	0/0	24/26 (92%)
Primary suture	0/0	25/31	0/0	25/31 (81%)
Secondary suture	9/7	12/8	3/5	18/26 (70%)
Secondary graft	22/17	21/40	25/56	63/118 (53%)
Total elements	48/57	54/83	28/61	130/201 (65%)

Results are given as number of elements/total elements recovering to grade 3 or better (LSUHSC system). Primary = repair within 72 hours of injury; secondary = delayed repair, usually after several weeks.

[a] N = 71.

acutely, end-to-end suture repair was usually possible and gave very good results. Blunt injuries had delayed repair so that the extent of trimming necessary to reach healthy tissue could be determined. Grafts therefore were usually necessary. Outcomes with blunt injuries were less favorable than with sharp injuries because these were more serious, with longitudinal injury more likely requiring grafts for repair rather than end-to-end suture. This series and the GSW series show that overall results are better with end-to-end suture than with graft repairs provided the circumstances are right so that this procedure can be performed without undue tension.

Despite a potentially transecting mechanism, some elements even with severe or complete loss in their distribution preoperatively were in continuity. They were managed, when possible, like other presumed plexus lesions in continuity by NAP recordings across the lesion; based on NAP findings, they were treated with either neurolysis or resection and repair. The latter was usually treated by grafts or less frequently by suture. If NAPs were recorded across the lesion, only a neurolysis was performed. The outcome in this subset of lesions in continuity associated with lacerating injury was favorable, with 47 of 58 elements recovering to grade 3 or better function.

Gunshot wounds

An analysis of the plexus lesions injured by GSW was also interesting. Table 3 shows the large role played by graft repair. Again, less favorable elements for repair are grouped together with those more favorable for repair. End-to-end suture was superior in terms of restitution to grade 3 or better function in 19 of 27 elements (70%) versus grafts in 75 of 138 elements (54%). This finding

showed that grafts were necessary in lengthier and thus more severe injuries, but again, if circumstances permitted, outcomes with end-to-end suture were superior to those with graft repair. NAP recording was extremely important in this group of patients because 46 of 202 (20%) elements, which were believed to have complete loss by clinical and EMG criteria preoperatively, transmitted operative NAPs across their lesion, indicating regeneration; therefore, these elements could receive neurolysis only with the expected good results. Of equal importance, nine elements believed to have incomplete injury did not transmit an NAP, and these had repair by either suture (six cases) or graft (three cases). Variations in anatomy found at the time of operation, particularly for some infraclavicular GSW injuries, accounted for most of these latter discrepancies.

The best results with grafts were for C5, C6, and upper trunk lesions, but also for C7 and middle trunk injuries. At an infraclavicular level,

Table 3
Surgical outcome in gunshot wound injuries[a]

Type of lesion	Neurolysis (+NAPs)	Suture	Graft
Elements with complete loss (202 elements)	42/46 (91%)	14/21 (67%)	73/135 (54%)
Elements with incomplete loss (91 elements)	78/82 (95%)	5/6 (83%)	2/3 (67%)
Total (293 elements)	120/128 (94%)	19/27 (70%)	75/138 (54%)

Results are given as number of elements/total elements recovering to grade 3 or better (see Box 1).

NAPs indicate increased conduction across a lesion in continuity.

[a] N = 118.

repairs of the lateral cord and its outflows and the posterior cord to the axillary nerve did well. Repairs of the posterior cord to the radial nerve did less well, however. Furthermore, repairs of the medial cord to the median nerve also did well. Repairs to the C8 T1 to lower trunk and medial cord and medial cord to ulnar did poorly unless partially injured or shown to be regenerating by NAP recordings.

Stretch/contusion injuries

Earlier, before the authors began to add transfers to their armamentarium for repair of stretch injures, they would try for direct repair of as many elements as possible but would also use descending cervical plexus as a transfer but not accessory, medial pectoral branches or intercostals until later in the series. Figs. 1 through 3 depict the use of NAP recordings and some of the resultant direct repairs on C5, C6 (C7) cases.

Tables 4 through 6 show outcomes using grafts for direct plexus repair for various stretch/contusion patterns. Descending cervical plexus also had

been used to add to the direct repairs in 13% of the C5 and C6 repairs and 27% of the C5, C6, and C7 repairs. Tables 4 and 5, which summarize outcomes for C5/C6 and C5, C6, and C7 stretches, show how the pattern of avulsions and whether they affected C5 or C6 or both changed outcomes. The additional value of transfer of accessory for shoulder and medial pectoral or other transfer for biceps in a smaller cohort of patients operated on between 1998 and 2000 can be seen by these tables. Nonetheless, it can also be appreciated that direct repairs by grafts had much to offer.

Since 2000, the authors have added transfers to most direct plexus repairs for stretch injuries. Accessory has been transferred to suprascapular nerve unless there is evidence of regeneration to it or C5 is usable as a lead-out for grafts. When this has been the case, most of the C5 grafts usually have been led to the posterior division of upper trunk. The authors favor, when possible, for C5, C6, and C7 stretch injuries, the use of medial pectoral branches to add to any direct repair they gain for elements leading to musculocutaneous

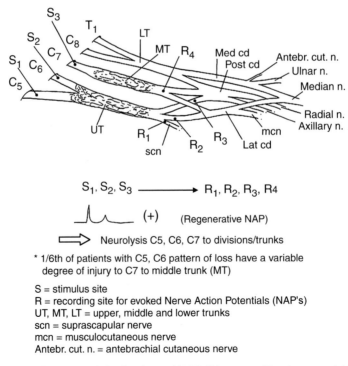

$$S_1, S_2, S_3 \longrightarrow R_1, R_2, R_3, R4$$

(+)   (Regenerative NAP)

⇒ Neurolysis C5, C6, C7 to divisions/trunks

* 1/6th of patients with C5, C6 pattern of loss have a variable degree of injury to C7 to middle trunk (MT)

S = stimulus site
R = recording site for evoked Nerve Action Potentials (NAP's)
UT, MT, LT = upper, middle and lower trunks
scn = suprascapular nerve
mcn = musculocutaneous nerve
Antebr. cut. n. = antebrachial cutaneous nerve

Fig. 1. C5, C6 (C7) pattern of loss. One sixth of patients with C5, C6 pattern of loss have a variable degree of injury to C7 to middle trunk (MT). Antebr. cut. n., antebrachial cutaneous nerve; Lat cd, lateral cord; LT, lower trunk; Med cd, medial cord; mcn, musculocutaneous nerve; Post cd, posterior cord; R, recording site for evoked NAPs; S, stimulus site; scn, suprascapular nerve; UT, upper trunk.

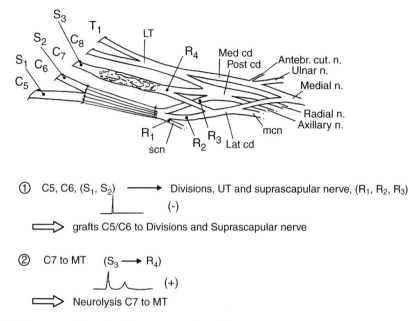

① C5, C6, (S$_1$, S$_2$) ⟶ Divisions, UT and suprascapular nerve, (R$_1$, R$_2$, R$_3$)

(-)

⟹ grafts C5/C6 to Divisions and Suprascapular nerve

② C7 to MT (S$_3$ ⟶ R$_4$)

(+)

⟹ Neurolysis C7 to MT

Fig. 2. C5, C6 (C7) pattern of loss. Antebr. cut. n., antebrachial cutaneous nerve; Lat cd, lateral cord; LT, lower trunk; Med cd, medial cord; mcn, musculocutaneous nerve; MT, middle trunk; Post cd, posterior cord; R, recording site for evoked NAPs; S, stimulus site; scn, suprascapular nerve; UT, upper trunk.

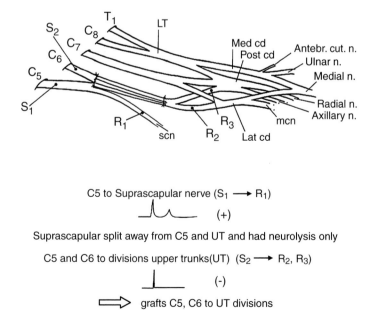

C5 to Suprascapular nerve (S$_1$ ⟶ R$_1$)

(+)

Suprascapular split away from C5 and UT and had neurolysis only

C5 and C6 to divisions upper trunks(UT) (S$_2$ ⟶ R$_2$, R$_3$)

(-)

⟹ grafts C5, C6 to UT divisions

Fig. 3. C5, C6 (C7) pattern of loss. Antebr. cut. n., antebrachial cutaneous nerve; Lat cd, lateral cord; LT, lower trunk; Med cd, medial cord; mcn, musculocutaneous nerve; MT, middle trunk; Post cd, posterior cord; R, recording site for evoked NAPs; S, stimulus site; scn, suprascapular nerve; UT, upper trunk.

Table 4
Operative results of C5, C6 stretch injuries with complete loss

Operation	No. patients (N = 55)	Results (averaged)
Grafts C5, C6	34	Grade 3 = 12; grade 3–4 = 7; grade 4 = 8
C5 grafts, C6 avulsed, descending[a]	5	Cervical plexus used grade 2–3
C5 avulsed, C6 grafts, descending cervical plexus used[b]	2	Grade 3–4
Neurolysis of C5 and C6 (positive NAPs)	12	Grade 3–4
C5 neurolysis, C6 grafts	2	Grade 3–4

[a] These cases might have done better had medial pectoral branch transfer to musculocutaneous nerve been added. Four cases done between 1998 and 2000 in this fashion had averaged outcomes of 4.

[b] These cases might have done better had accessory nerve transfer to suprascapular nerve been added. Two cases done between 1998 and 2000 in this fashion had averaged outcomes of 3.8.

Table 5
Operative results of C5, C6 and C7 stretch injuries with complete loss

Operation	No. patients (N = 75)	Results (averaged)
Grafts of C5, C6 and C7	31	Grade ≥3–4
C5 grafts, C6 and C7 avulsed, descending cervical plexus used[a]	10	Grade 2–3
C5 and C6 grafts, C7 avulsed, descending plexus used	10	Grade 3
C5 avulsed, C6 and C7 grafts, descending plexus used[b]	6	Grade 3–4
Neurolysis C5, C6 and C7 (positive NAPs)	18	Grade 4

[a] These cases might have done better had medial pectoral branch transfer to musculocutaneous nerve been added. Three cases done between 1998 and 2000 in this fashion had averaged outcome of 3.7.

[b] These cases might have done better had distal accessory nerve been transferred to suprascapular nerve as an additional step. Two cases done between 1998 and 2000 in this fashion had averaged outcome of 3.5.

nerve. Figs. 4 through 6 depict the use of nerve transfers to bolster potential outcomes from direct repairs in patients with C5, C6 (C7) patterns of loss.

Recently, one of the current authors (R.L.T.) has begun to use the Oberlin transfer of a fascicle of the ulnar nerve to the musculocutaneous nerve. This experience, although encouraging, is too nascent to report, but others have found this to be a favorable transfer. When there has been proximal direct repair with possible lead-in to musculocutaneous nerve, the latter is split in

a longitudinal direction. One distal half is then used for lead-in from medial pectoral branches or ulnar nerve, whereas the other half is left intact to receive proximal down-flow. If possible, either transfer is done without an intervening graft because the use of an intervening graft seems to decrease results. This type of "pants-over-vest" approach seems to make sense because it at least theoretically maximizes the number of axons brought to bear on a denervated structure.

Table 6
Overall postoperative grades on patients with supraclavicular plexus stretch injuries patients[a]

Initial loss	Postoperative grade									Totals
	0	1	1–2	2	2–3	3	3–4	4	4–5	
C5/C6 (C)	1	0	0	0	6	14	18	9	7	55
C5/C6/C7 (C)	1	0	0	2	14	23	20	9	6	75
C5 to T1 (C)	21	8	15	29	62	40	20	13	0	208
C5 to C8 (C)	0	0	0	0	0	1	1	0	0	2
C6/C7/C8/T1 (C)	0	0	0	1	0	2	1	0	0	4
C7 to T1 (C)	0	0	0	0	1	1	0	0	0	2
C8 to T1 (C)	2	3	2	2	0	2	0	0	0	11
C8 to T1 (I)	0	0	0	0	0	0	2	2	3	7
C7/C8/T1 (I)	0	0	0	0	0	1	1	0	0	2
Total	25	11	17	34	83	84	63	33	16	366

C = complete or nearly complete loss; I = incomplete loss.
[a] N = 366.

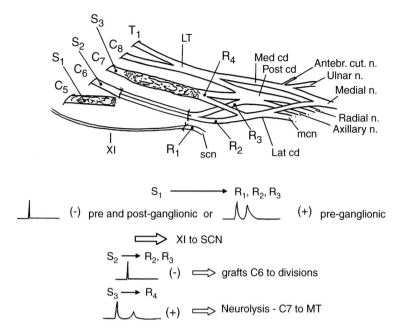

Fig. 4. C5, C6 (C7) pattern of loss. Antebr. cut. n., antebrachial cutaneous nerve; Lat cd, lateral cord; LT, lower trunk; Med cd, medial cord; mcn, musculocutaneous nerve; MT, middle trunk; Post cd, posterior cord; R, recording site for evoked NAPs; S, stimulus site; scn/SCN, suprascapular nerve; UT, upper trunk.

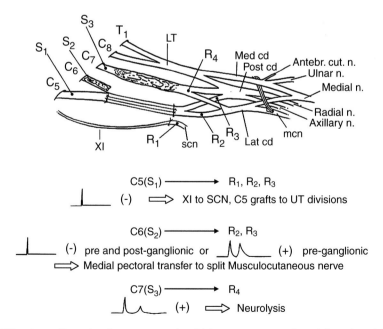

Fig. 5. C5, C6 (C7) pattern of loss. Antebr. cut. n., antebrachial cutaneous nerve; Lat cd, lateral cord; LT, lower trunk; Med cd, medial cord; mcn, musculocutaneous nerve; MT, middle trunk; Post cd, posterior cord; R, recording site for evoked NAPs; S, stimulus site; scn/SCN, suprascapular nerve; UT, upper trunk.

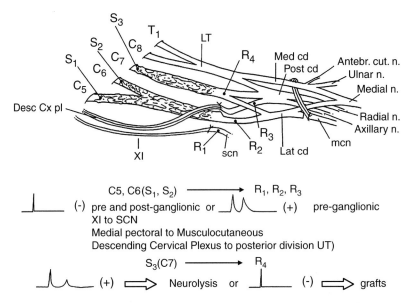

Fig. 6. C5, C6 (C7) pattern of loss. Antebr. cut. n., antebrachial cutaneous nerve; Desc Cx pl, descending cervical plexus; Lat cd, lateral cord; LT, lower trunk; Med cd, medial cord; mcn, musculocutaneous nerve; MT, middle trunk; Post cd, posterior cord; R, recording site for evoked NAPs; S, stimulus site; scn/SCN, suprascapular nerve; UT, upper trunk.

Table 6 gives the postoperative grades for stretch injuries with various preoperative distributions. Almost all of the data in this table on flail arms come from direct graft repair. The difficulties in obtaining satisfactory results in the flail arm (C5 to T1 loss) where loss is complete are evident. It is also evident that outcomes with direct repair of many stretch injuries are less than optimal. This situation has prompted the current authors to add nerve transfers to direct repair whenever possible in recent years.

In patients with C5-6 stretch injuries, medial pectoral nerve transfer added to musculocutaneous nerve improved grades to an average of 4. Accessory to suprascapular transfers improved the grade in that subset of patients to 3.8 (see Table 4).

In patients with C5, C6, and C7 stretch injuries, medial pectoral transfer to musculocutaneous nerve helped achieve an average grade of 3.7, whereas XI (necessary nerve) to suprascapular nerve improved average grades to 3.5 (see Table 5).

Since 1998, another hundred or so patients have had nerve transfers added to whatever direct repair the authors could obtain. Detailed outcomes of these patients will be the subject of another article, but experience to date with such an approach has been encouraging.

In the C5, C6 or C5, C6 and C7 cases, accessory has been placed to suprascapular and usually medial pectoral branches to a split half of the musculocutaneous nerve. Direct graft repairs, when possible because of sufficient lead-out, usually have been placed to the divisions of upper and, if possible, middle trunks.

In the flail arm cases in which medial pectoral or other nerves are not available for transfer, intercostal nerves have been transferred end-to-end to musculocutaneous nerve, which has been sectioned proximally and then curved down distally to meet the intercostals at the level of the axilla. The accessory nerve has been mobilized so that it can be sutured directly to the suprascapular nerve, which, whenever possible, is sectioned well proximally. Any available direct outflow from C5, and less frequently C6 and rarely C7, has been led to the posterior division of the upper trunk, posterior cord, or the portion of lateral cord going to the median nerve. When direct repair of C6 outflow is judged to be feasible, the musculocutaneous nerve is split longitudinally so that intercostals are sewn into one half of the nerve. Figs. 7 through 10 depict some of the repairs used in the patients with flail arms.

Discussion

Open injuries

The direct repair of plexus elements injured by lacerations and GSWs is not only possible but

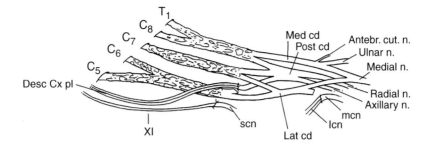

All 5 spinal nerves with either pre and post-gangliotic
injury or pre-gangliotic injury ⇒

XI to Suprascapular nerve
Intercostal nerves(ICN) to Musculocutaneous nerve
Descending Cervical Plexus to posterior division or uper trunk

Fig. 7. C5 through T1 loss (flail arm). Antebr. cut. n., antebrachial cutaneous nerve; Desc Cx pl, descending cervical plexus; Icn, intercostal nerve; Lat cd, lateral cord; Med cd, medial cord; mcn, musculocutaneous nerve; Post cd, posterior cord; scn, suprascapular nerve.

gives acceptable results. End-to-end repair is usually, although not always, possible for most transections caused by laceration or GSWs. Where either mechanism gives lesions in continuity, results with direct repair, usually by grafts, is also acceptable. These results are possible if intraoperative electrophysiologic studies (usually NAP recordings) are used to differentiate those lesions not needing repair from those that do. It is possible

that the addition of nerve transfers under certain circumstances might add to these outcomes, but the authors have had limited experience with such repairs in these injury categories.

Lacerations

The advantages of relatively acute repair for sharply transected elements are evident in the data

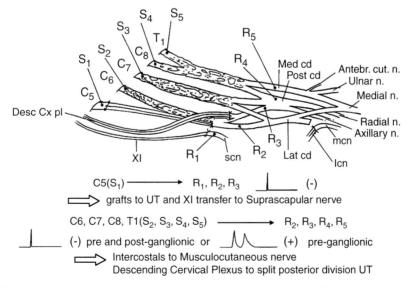

$C5(S_1)$ ⟶ R_1, R_2, R_3 ⊥ (-)
⇒ grafts to UT and XI transfer to Suprascapular nerve

$C6, C7, C8, T1(S_2, S_3, S_4, S_5)$ ⟶ R_2, R_3, R_4, R_5

⊥ (-) pre and post-ganglionic or /\\ (+) pre-ganglionic
⇒ Intercostals to Musculocutaneous nerve
Descending Cervical Plexus to split posterior division UT

Fig. 8. Another pattern of C5 through T1 loss (flail arm). Antebr. cut. n., antebrachial cutaneous nerve; Desc Cx pl, descending cervical plexus; Icn, intercostal nerve; Lat cd, lateral cord; Med cd, medial cord; mcn, musculocutaneous nerve; Post cd, posterior cord; R, recording site for evoked NAPs; S, stimulus site; scn, suprascapular nerve; UT, upper trunk.

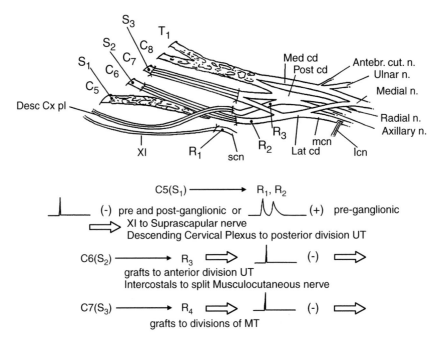

Fig. 9. C5 through T1 loss (flail arm). Antebr. cut. n., antebrachial cutaneous nerve; Desc Cx pl, descending cervical plexus; Icn, intercostal nerve; Lat cd, lateral cord; Med cd, medial cord; mcn, musculocutaneous nerve; MT, middle trunk; Post cd, posterior cord; R, recording site for evoked NAPs; S, stimulus site; scn, suprascapular nerve; UT, upper trunk.

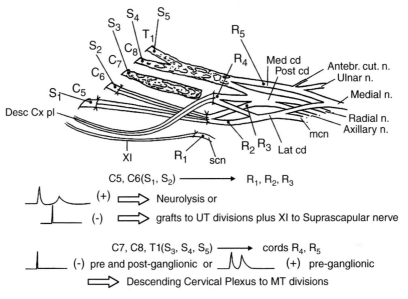

Fig. 10. C5 through T1 loss (flail arm). Antebr. cut. n., antebrachial cutaneous nerve; Desc Cx pl, descending cervical plexus; Lat cd, lateral cord; Med cd, medial cord; mcn, musculocutaneous nerve; MT, middle trunk; Post cd, posterior cord; R, recording site for evoked NAPs; S, stimulus site; scn, suprascapular nerve; UT, upper trunk.

presented, because end-to-end repair is more likely under these circumstances than had repair been delayed. Transection by blunt mechanisms was managed by delayed repair so that resection to relatively healthy tissue could be done. Despite laceration as a mechanism of injury, some elements with loss in their distribution had lesions in continuity. NAP recordings were used on these elements to determine the need for resection and then end-to-end suture or a graft was done for those elements without NAPs across their lesions.

Gunshot wounds

Some gunshot injuries involving the plexus improve enough in the early months so that surgery on the plexus is not needed [12,13]. Only 15% of the serious injuries transect one or more plexus elements, so lesions in continuity are the most common pathology. NAP recordings then play an important role in determining the need for resection and direct repair. Thus, 46 of 202 elements (23%) with complete loss clinically by EMG at 3 or more months post injury transmitted an NAP and were regenerating. One hundred fifty-six other injured elements did not transmit an NAP and had direct repair either by end-to-end suture or by grafts. Most of the 91 elements believed to have incomplete loss preoperatively transmitted NAPs and had neurolysis, but importantly, nine elements did not and they required repair.

Stretch/contusion injuries, including avulsions

Operative inspection of the injured portion of the supraclavicular plexus is also important in patients with flail arm (C5–T1). A group of 208 patients with flail arm underwent preoperative clinical observation and myelographic examination and EMG workup of each root, matched with results of operative inspection of spinal nerves and plexus elements [14]. Of 1040 root levels studied, 470 had irreparable proximal spinal nerve or nerve root lesions. Approximately 35% of the avulsions involved C7, C8, and T1. Another 35% involved C7 and C8, whereas 20% had other combinations, which included C6. Only 4% of patients had avulsion of all five levels, including C5, and only 10% of patients had avulsion of C5 as part of the pattern of loss. Thus, repairs, usually by grafts, were possible in about half of the levels inspected. Grafts were often long, so good or better results were only achieved in 35%. Nonetheless, it was shown that direct repair was feasible in some patients and gave good results, especially if C5

and C6 were usable for outflow. In the patients with flail arm, C5 can frequently and C6 can sometimes be a source of fascicular lead-out for direct repair by grafts and should be inspected and tested in most cases.

Outcomes in C5, C6, and C7 lesions, although acceptable before 1998, have improved since then by the addition of nerve transfers. This situation also is true for patients with flail arm (C5 to T1). Recovery of proximal shoulder and upper arm function was acceptable but forearm recovery was poor or nonexistent, so the overall grade for recovery in the C5, C6, and C7 distribution in the flail arm limbs with direct repairs was only grade 3 in 35% of patients. When transfers were added to direct repair of one or more spinal nerve levels, 45% of patients achieved an LSUHSC grade 3 or better level. Furthermore, where only transfers without direct repair were done, usually for C5 through T1 avulsions, grade 3 or better levels were only achieved in 30% of patients.

Shoulder abduction

Shoulder abduction is one of the two most necessary proximal functions for a useful arm. Initiation of abduction is most important and that is provided by the supraspinatus for the first 30° to 40°. External rotation of the shoulder is also important and that is provided by infraspinatus. Therefore, neurotization of the suprascapular nerve is a high priority with stretch/contusive plexus injuries. The use of the accessory nerve to do this was devised some years ago and has proved effective, especially if transferred end to end rather than with the interposition of grafts [15–18].

Elbow flexion

Of equal importance to usable function is the restoration of elbow flexion. This result can be achieved in some patients with supraclavicular stretch injuries by direct repair using grafts, even though these grafts are several inches long. Neurotization by nerve transfer more frequently produces usable elbow flexion [19,20], especially if C8-T1 and its outflows are functional, because then either the medial pectoral branches or fasicles of the ulnar nerve can be transferred to the musculocutaneous nerve [21]. Both methods can be effective, although proponents of the Oberlin technique prefer it because placement of an ulnar fasicle into the motor portion of the musculocutaneous nerve is more selective [22]. If C8-T1 and its outflows are damaged, as they are in patients with flail arm, then either intercostal transfers or the use of contralateral C7 has been recommended. The original intercostal transfers were done with the help of interposed grafts [23–26]. Experience has shown that intercostals placed directly to musculocutaneous nerve provide more frequent and better results than those with interposed grafts [27–29].

Other transfers

The current authors have not routinely used phrenic nerve as a source of axons for transfer, although others have had good results [30]. In the authors' experience, the loss of phrenic function during supraclavicular brachial plexus dissections is not without secondary complications, such as atelectasis and pneumonia and occasional complaints from patients about shortness of breath. The authors therefore have not purposely sectioned this nerve for transfer nor have they taken the chance, admittedly small, of endangering function of the contralateral limb by using contralateral C7 as a source of axons. Unless the operation is performed at the level of the spinal canal, the use of C7 for outflow to neurotize contralateral plexus nerves also requires relatively lengthy grafts [31]. Although they have fewer motor fibers than accessory or contralateral C7, the C3, C4 spinal nerves or their outflows are also a nonplexus source of axons [32–34]. Thus, the descending cervical plexus can provide some fibers to either the upper or middle trunk posterior division to the posterior cord. If some direct lead-out

to the posterior divisions by direct repair is possible, then the descending plexus can be placed to the anterior division of the middle trunk.

Direct repair supplemented by transfers

When some direct repair is possible, the current authors have tried to preserve routes for down-flow to more distal plexus elements, and especially the musculocutaneous nerve, by splitting them longitudinally and placing the transferred nerve into half of the recipient nerve rather than into the whole element or nerve. This approach has been done most often after direct repair of one or more proximal elements leading to the musculocutaneous nerve. The musculocutaneous nerve is then split longitudinally and one half is anastomosed to the medial pectoral branches and the other half is left alone for receipt of any down-flow from the proximal repair. When the thoracodorsal nerve can be transferred into the axillary nerve to provide some recovery of the deltoid muscle, it has been done to half of the recipient nerve [35]. This approach works best if

---

Box 2. Repair preference for C5/C6 stretch or C5/C6/C7 stretch injuries

1. Neurolysis if NAPs indicate regeneration
2. Direct repair if NAPs are negative (flat) and proximal fascicular structure is found on sectioning spinal nerve plus addition of medial pectoral to split musculocutaneous nerve (for C6 avulsion) or accessory to suprascapular nerve (for C5 avulsion)
3. Accessory and medial pectoral transfers and, less frequently, descending cervical plexus transfers if NAP studies indicate preganglionic lesion or sectioning indicates pre- and postganglionic lesions of C5 and C6.

Box 3. Repair preferences for C5 through T1 stretch injuries or flail arm

1. Neurolysis where NAPs indicate regeneration. (This finding is infrequent but does occur.)
2. Direct repair if NAPs are negative and yet, on sectioning, fascicular structure is found proximally. Grafts are from proximal spinal nerves to divisions or cords. Added in are the following: (1) accessory to suprascapular nerve, (2) descending cervical plexus to posterior division of upper trunk or middle trunk and its divisions, (3) intercostals (three or four) to a longitudinally split portion of musculocutaneous nerve.
3. If all five plexus roots are avulsed, the following repairs are preferred: (1) XI (necessary nerve) to suprascapular nerve, (2) intercostal nerves to musculocutaneous nerve, and (3) either descending cervical plexus or XI input to sternocleidomastoid muscle placed to posterior division of upper trunk.

Table 7
Surgical outcome in infraclavicular plexus stretch injuries[a]

Plexus elements	No. elements (average grade of recovery achieved)			
	Neurolysis[b]	Suture	Grafts	Split repair
Cords				
Lateral	12 (4.5)	3 (4.3)	6 (3.8)	3 (4)
Medial	16 (3.9)	2 (2.2)	7 (1.2)	4 (3.6)
Posterior	14 (4.1)	2 (3.6)	6 (3.0)	3 (3.5)
Cords to nerves				
Lateral to musculocutaneous	20 (4.4)	0 (0)	35 (3.8)	0 (0)
Lateral to median	29 (4.1)	1 (4)	19 (3)	0 (0)
Medial to median	24 (4.3)	1 (4)	17 (3)	0 (0)
Medial to ulnar	33 (3.6)	1 (0)	13 (1.4)	1 (2.3)
Posterior to radial	29 (4.1)	1 (0)	32 (2.7)	3 (3.5)
Posterior to axillary	28 (4.7)	1 (3)	48 (3.5)	1 (4)
Totals				
Elements/results	205 (4.2)	12 (2.3)	183 (2.8)	15 (3.6)

[a] N = 143.
[b] Neurolysis based on a positive NAP.

some down-flow to the axillary nerve can be gained by more direct repair proximally, such as C5 by means of grafts to the posterior division of the upper trunk. This approach has not been used with the suprascapular nerve, which is either repaired directly by grafts from C5 and C6 or by neurotization through transfer of accessory to the nerve without other input.

To date, this "pants-over-vest" approach has paid dividends, although outcomes still leave much to be desired in this difficult category of injury, especially for the patients with flail arm for whom eventual usefulness of the limb may be quite limited [36,37]. The authors' current preferences for repair of C5-6, C5, C6, C7, and C5 through T1 (flail arm) stretch injuries are outlined in Boxes 2 and 3.

Infraclavicular stretch injuries

Although some infraclavicular stretch injuries improve spontaneously, many do not and require surgery for correction [38].

Most of the infraclavicular stretch injuries managed before and since 1998 in this series had direct repair rather than nerve transfers. Outcomes were best for lateral and posterior cord lesions and their outflows. Medial cord to median repair also gave good results (Table 7).

Other techniques

The current authors applaud the concepts but do not at this time perform other more recently described reconstructive techniques, such as neurotized and vascularized free-muscle transfers for plexus stretch/contusion/avulsive lesions [39]. They also have not undertaken spinal cord implantation for avulsed roots and prefer to await more definitive data about outcomes and possible spinal cord complications [40]. Certainly, various repair techniques will continue to evolve, especially for the supraclavicular stretch palsies needing reconstruction [41–43].

References

[1] Merrell G, Barrie K, Katz D, Wolfe S. Results of nerve transfer for restoration of shoulder and elbow function in the context of a meta-analysis of the English literature. J Hand Surg 2001;26A(2):303–14.
[2] Kline D, Hudson A. Lacerations to brachial plexus. In: Nerve injuries: operative results for major nerve injuries, entrapments, and tumors. Philadelphia: WB Saunders; 1995. p. 371–80.
[3] Kline D. Civilian gunshot wounds to the brachial plexus. J Neurosurg 1989;70:166–74.
[4] Birch R, Bonney G, Wynn Parry CB. Surgical disorders of peripheral nerves. New York: Churchill Livingstone; 1998.
[5] Seddon H. Surgical disorders of the peripheral nerves. Edinburgh, UK: E & S Livingston; 1972.
[6] Simesen K, Haase J. Microsurgery in brachial plexus lesions. Acta Orthop Scand 1985;56:238–41.
[7] Sunderland S. Nerve injuries and their repairs. A critical appraisal. Edinburgh, UK: Churchill Livingstone; 1991.
[8] Friedman AH. Neurotization of elements of the brachial plexus. Neurosurg Clin N Am 1991;2:165–74.

[9] Kim D, Cho Y, Tiel R, Kline D. Outcomes in surgery in 1019 brachial plexus lesions treated at LSUHSC. J Neurosurg 2003;53(5):1005–16.

[10] Landi A, Copeland SA, Wynn Parry CB, Jones SJ. The role of somatosensory evoked potentials and nerve conduction studies in the surgical management of brachial plexus injuries. J Bone Joint Surg 1980; 62N:492–6.

[11] Millesi H. Surgical management of brachial plexus injuries. J Hand Surg 1977;2:367–79.

[12] Nulsen FE, Slade HW. Recovery following injury to the brachial plexus. In: Woodhall B, Beebe GW, editors. Peripheral nerve regeneration: a follow-up study of 3,656 World War II injuries. Washington, DC: US Government Printing Office; 1957. p. 389–408.

[13] Omer G. Results of untreated peripheral nerve injuries. Clin Orthop Rel Res 1982;163:15–9.

[14] Kline D, Hudson A. Stretch injuries to brachial plexus. In: Nerve injuries: operative results of major nerve inures, entrapments, and tumors. Philadelphia: WB Saunders; 1995. p. 397–460.

[15] Allieu U, Cenac P. Neurotization via the spinal accessory nerve incomplete paralysis due to multiple avulsion injuries of the brachial plexus. Clin Orthop 1988;237:67–74.

[16] Samardzic M, Grujicic D, Antunovic V. Nerve transfer in brachial plexus traction injuries. J Neurosurg 1992;76:191–7.

[17] Narakas AO. Neurotization in the treatment of brachial plexus injuries. In: Gelberman RH, editor. Operative nerve repair and reconstruction. Philadelphia: JB Lippincott; 1991. p. 1329–58.

[18] Chuang DC-C, Lee GW, Hashem F, Wei F-C. Restoration of shoulder abduction by nerve transfer in avulsion brachial plexus injury: evaluation of 99 patients with various nerve transfers. Plast Reconstr Surg 1995;96:122–8.

[19] Sedel L. Repair of severe traction lesions of the brachial plexus. Clin Orthop 1988;237:62–6.

[20] Terzis JK, Vekris MD, Soucacos PN. Outcomes of brachial plexus reconstruction in 204 patients with devastating paralysis. Plast Reconstr Surg 1999; 104:1221–40.

[21] Brandt KE, Mackinnon SE. A technique for maximizing biceps recovery in brachial plexus reconstruction. J Hand Surg 1993;18A:726–33.

[22] Oberlin C, Beal D, Leechavengvongs S, Salon A, Dauge MC, Sarcy JJ. Nerve transfer to biceps muscle using a part of ulnar nerve for C5–C6 avulsion of the brachial plexus: anatomical study and report of four cases. J Hand Surg 1994;19A: 232–7.

[23] Tsuyama N, Hara T. Intercostal nerve transfer in the treatment of brachial plexus injury of root-avulsion type. Orthopaedic surgery and traumatology. In: Proceedings of the 12th Congress, Tel Aviv. New York: Elsevier; 1972. p. 351–3.

[24] Ploncard P. A new approach to the intercosto-brachial anastomosis in the treatment of brachial plexus paralysis due to root avulsion. Late results. Acta Neurochir 1982;61:281–90.

[25] Narakas A. Brachial plexus surgery. Orthop Clin N Am 1981;12:303–23.

[26] Dolenc VV. Intercostal neurotization of the peripheral nerves in avulsion plexus injures. Clin Plast Surg 1984;11:143–7.

[27] Nagano A, Tsuyama N, Ochiai N, Hara T, Takahashi M. Direct nerve crossing with the intercostal nerve to treat avulsion injuries of the brachial plexus. J Hand Surg 1989;14A:980–5.

[28] Kanaya F, Gonzalez M, Park C-M, Kutz JE, Kleinert He, Tsai T-M. Improvement in motor function after brachial plexus surgery. J Hand Surg 1990;15A: 30–6.

[29] Malessy M, Thomeer R. Evaluation of intercostal to musculocutaneous nerve transfer in reconstructive brachial plexus surgery. J Neurosurg 1998;88: 266–71.

[30] Gu Y-D, Wu M-M, Zhen Y-L, et al. Phrenic nerve transfer for treatment of root avulsion of the brachial plexus. Chin Med J 1990;103:267–70.

[31] Gu Y-D, Chen D-S, Zhang G-M, et al. Long-term functional results of contralateral C7 transfer. J Reconstr Microsurg 1998;12:57–9.

[32] Brunelli G. Neurotization of avulsed roots of the brachial plexus by means of anterior nerves of the cervical plexus. In: Terzis JK, editor. Microconstruction of nerve injuries. Philadelphia: WB Saunders; 1987. p. 435–45.

[33] Rutowski R. Neurotizations by means of the cervical plexus in over 100 patients with from one to five root avulsions of the brachial plexus. Microsurgery 1993; 14:285–8.

[34] Yamada S, Lonser RR, Iacono RP, Morenski JD, Bailey L. Bypass coaptation procedures for cervical nerve root avulsion. Neurosurgery 1996;38: 1145–52.

[35] Dai S-Y, Lin D-X, Han Z, Zhoug S-Z. Transference of thoracodorsal nerve to musculocutaneous or axillary nerve in old traumatic injury. J Hand Surg 1990; 15A:36–7.

[36] Hentz VR, Narakas A. The results of microneurosurgical reconstruction in complete brachial plexus palsy. Orthop Clin North Am 1988;19: 107–14.

[37] Choi PD, Novak CB, Mackinnon SE, Kline DG. Quality of life and functional outcome following brachial plexus injury. J Hand Surg 1997;22: 605–12.

[38] Leffert R, Seddon H. Infraclavicular brachial plexus injuries. J Bone Joint Surg [Br] 1965;47:9–22.

[39] Doi K, Sakai K, Kunata N. Double-muscle technique for reconstruction of prehension after complete avulsion of brachial plexus. J Hand Surg 1995;20A:408–14.

[40] Carlsted T, Anand P, Hallin R, Misra PV, Norem G, Seferlis T. Spinal nerve root repair and reimplantation of avulsed ventral roots into the spinal cord after brachial plexus injury. J Neurosurg 2000;93: 237–47.

[41] Berger A, Becker MH-J. Brachial plexus surgery: our concept of the last twelve years. Microsurgery 1994;15:760–7.

[42] Waikakul S, Wongtragul S, Vanadurongwan V. Restoration of elbow flexion in brachial plexus avulsion injury: comparing spinal accessory nerve transfer with intercostal nerve transfer. J Hand Surg 1999; 24A:571–7.

[43] Spinner R, Kline D. Surgery for peripheral nerve and brachial plexus injures or other nerve lesions. Muscle Nerve 2000;23:680–97.

Nerve Transfers in Adult Brachial Plexus Injuries: My Methods

David Chwei-Chin Chuang, MD

Department of Plastic Surgery, Chang Gung University Hospital, 199 Tun Hwa North Road,
Taipei-Linkou, Taipei (105), Taiwan

Neurolysis, nerve repair, nerve grafts, nerve transfer, functioning free-muscle transfer, and pedicle muscle transfer are the main surgical procedures for brachial plexus reconstruction [1–7]. Among these, nerve transfer, or neurotization, is growing in importance and popularity [8–10]. This procedure is mainly indicated in root avulsion injury, in which the spinal nerve or its rootlets are avulsed from the spinal cord. Many adult brachial plexus injuries are closed or traction-type injuries in which 55% to 75% of nerves sustain preganglionic root injuries, or avulsions [1–5]. When spinal nerve root avulsion occurs in a brachial plexus injury, nerve transfers provide possibly the only chance to reinnervate the distal part of the avulsed brachial plexus. In a root avulsion injury, the proximal end is not found or not available. Nerve transfer is an intentional transfer of a functional but less important nerve to the distal, irreparable, but more important, denervated avulsed nerve within the golden period (within 5 months after injury) after the injury. One or more nerve transfers are often used for shoulder, elbow, or hand function.

Nerve transfer, or neurotization, includes three major categories: extraplexal neurotization, intraplexal neurotization, and end-to-side (ETS) neurorrhaphy.

Extraplexal neurotization

Extraplexal neurotization is the transfer of a nonbrachial plexus component nerve to the brachial plexus for neurotization of an avulsed nerve. Sources commonly used include the phrenic

[11], spinal accessory [12], intercostal [13], deep cervical motor branches [14], hypoglossal [15], and contralateral C7 [16] transfers (Fig. 1). Other donor nerves, less commonly used donor nerves include the greater occipital nerve, the ramus of the levator scapular, and contralateral pectoral nerves [8,9]. Most nerve transfers are for motor neurotization, and only a few for purely sensory function.

Intraplexal neurotization

Intraplexal neurotization is the transfer of a spinal nerve or more distal plexus component with intact spinal cord connections to a more important denervated nerve.

In most cases, a ruptured proximal nerve is used. Examples include connecting the proximal stump of C5 or C6 to the distal aspect of C8, lower trunk, or median nerve [3,4,8,9], or the use of a portion of a functional ulnar nerve to the musculocutaneous nerve [17]. Other less commonly performed transfers include direct transfer or grafts from the anterior thoracic nerve, long thoracic nerve, thoracodorsal nerve, inferior ramus of the subscapular nerve, or the ramus for levator scapulae. Neuromuscular neurotization (direct implantation of motor nerve fascicles into denervated muscle) may also be used from intraplexal sources [8–10].

End-to-side neurorrhaphy

ETS neurorrhaphy is the final kind of nerve transfer [18]. In this technique, the distal stump of an irreparably injured nerve is implanted into a healthy nerve without injuring the function of the healthy nerve. The method is mostly used for

E-mail address: deardavid@pchome.com.tw

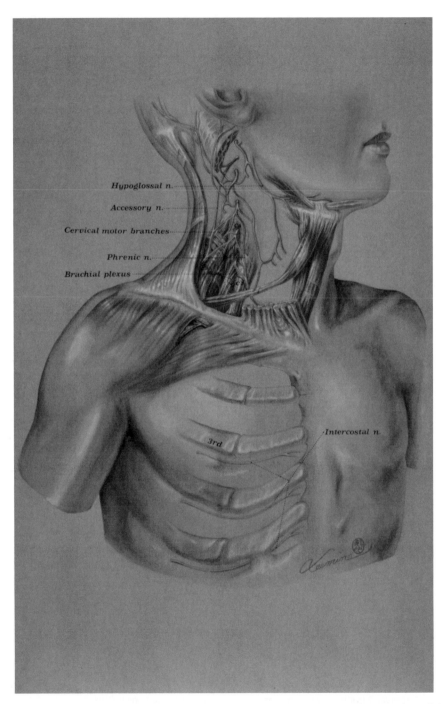

Fig. 1. Anatomic relationship of the available donor nerves for nerve transfer. n, nerve. (Illustration copyright Lee-Min Lee; with permission.)

sensory neurotization but, at present, is seldom used by most brachial plexus surgeons.

The numbers of myelinated axons in different donor nerves are listed in Table 1. These figures are based on studies by Narakas [19,20], Slingluff et al [21], Bonnel [22] and Bonnel and Rabischong [23], Terzis and Papakonstantinou [24], and others.

Table 1
Myelinated axon counts in donor nerves

Donor nerve	No. axons
C7	23,781 (mean, 16,000–40,000)
Hypoglossal	5000–6000
Phrenic	1756 (mean, ?800)
Spinal accessory	1500–1700 (or 2145)
Part of ulnar	1600
Long thoracic	1600–1800
One intercostal	800–1300
Deep cervical motor branches	893 (? 3400–4000)
Rami to the pectoral muscle	400–600/ramus

Materials and methods

Strict case inclusion criteria were used in this study. Two hundred thirty-three cases from the author's first 5 years of brachial plexus surgery were excluded (1985–1989) because of the immaturity of the surgeon. Surgeries performed after the year 2000 (259 cases) were excluded because of inadequate follow-up time (recovery from the contralateral C7 transfer usually takes at least 3 y to obtain results) [25]. Between 1990 and 2000, 773 patients with brachial plexus lesions were treated surgically. After excluding patients who had obstetric brachial plexus palsy (164 patients), thoracic outlet syndrome (27 patients), tumor of brachial plexus (16 patients), irradiation neuritis (6 patients), and brachial plexus poliolike neuritis (18 patients), 542 adult patients with brachial plexus injuries remained. Among these 542 patients, nerve transfers were used for functional restoration of the shoulder (266 patients), elbow function (301 patients), and hand or finger function (60 patients), and combined with functioning free-muscle transfer in 77 patients. Many patients had more than one such nerve transfer for simultaneous shoulder, elbow, or hand function.

General principles for nerve transfers

There is no generally agreed-on reconstructive algorithm for nerve transfer cases. Choices are made based on each surgeon's philosophy, knowledge, and experience. Patient-related factors are important as well, including elapsed time and severity of injury, age, and ability to cooperate with sometimes arduous rehabilitation. Finally, practicalities such as available facilities, equipment, and supplies, and availability of a knowledgeable and skilled rehabilitation therapist, are

important considerations. Nevertheless, the following general principles of nerve transfer surgery are applicable to most clinical settings:

1. Nerve reconstruction is almost always superior to palliative muscle or tendon transfer in adult brachial plexus injury if the nerve transfer gets good results. Adult brachial plexus injuries therefore should be explored in the early stage, within 5 months after injury [25–27]. Thereafter, the only late reconstructive options in a flail limb include tendon transfers [7,29], neurotized functioning free-muscle transfers [6,28] or functional muscle transfers [7,29,30].

2. In any nerve transfer, direct suture without tension is always superior to indirect suture with a nerve graft. This is especially true for the weak donor nerves such as intercostal nerves and the spinal accessory nerve. Lengthy dissection of both the donor and the recipient nerve may enable direct nerve coaptation.

3. Ipsilateral nerve transfer is always superior to the contralateral nerve transfer. For example, an ipsilateral C5 to median nerve transfer will be better than a contralateral C7 to median nerve transfer from the functional point of view (Figs. 2 and 3). The responsive motion shows faster and more powerfully in the ipsilateral nerve transfer than in the contralateral nerve transfer.

4. The health of the donor nerve is an important determining factor for success. For example, the success of the ipsilateral C5 transfer to the median nerve for hand function is usually determined by whether the proximal C5 stump is healthy.

5. The patient must be motivated and able to cooperate with surgical pre- and postoperative care recommendations. All patients undergoing neurotization need induction exercise or motivation exercise. For example, after intercostal or phrenic nerve transfer, patients will be directed to run, walk, or perform hill climbing to obtain deep breathing. As recovery progresses, frequent exercise of the reinnervated muscles provides an internal nerve impulse that is always superior to the external electric stimulation. Similarly, resistive range-of-motion shoulder exercises stimulating trapezius contraction ("move up or bend back" exercise) are important following surgery to re-educate spinal accessory

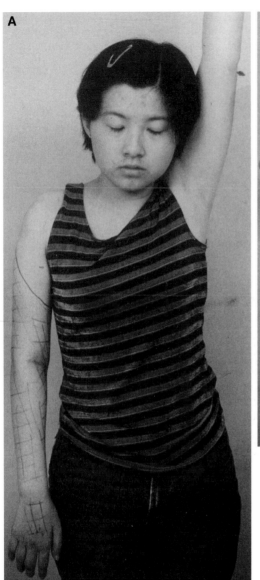
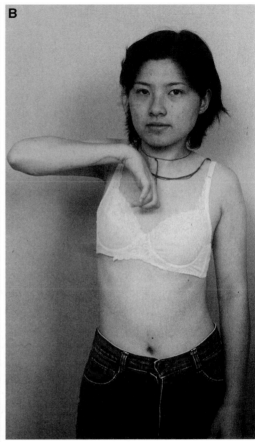

Fig. 2. (*A*) A 16-year-old girl sustained total root avulsion of the right brachial plexus with complete paralysis of the right upper limb. Results at 5 years after multiple nerve transfers: (*B*) spinal accessory nerve transfer to the suprascapular nerve for the shoulder; (*C*,*D*) three intercostal nerve transfer to the musculocutaneous nerve for elbow flexion; and (*E*–*G*) combined C5 and phrenic nerve transfers to the median nerve with a vascularized ulnar nerve graft for finger flexion, assisted by the use of an interphalangeal joint dynamic extension splint and thumb opposition splint (*F*). Four years after nerve reconstruction, the patient underwent a wrist arthrodesis and tendon transfers of the reinnervated flexor carpi radialis and palmaris longus to the fourth and fifth flexor digitorum profundus (FDP) to enhance finger flexion (*G*).

nerve transfers, as are tongue-to–hard palate push-up exercises in hypoglossal nerve transfer and grasp exercises of the donor extremity hand against resistance in contralateral C7 transfer. These exercises are called induction

exercises because they cause the transferred nerve to fire, stimulating contraction of the reinnervated muscle to contract.

6. In general, phrenic nerve transfers are most useful for shoulder function or arm extensors,

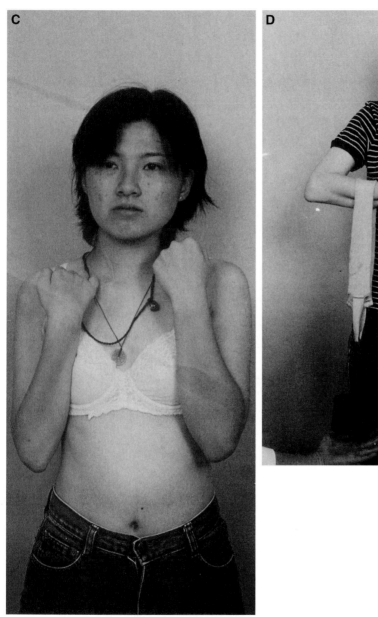

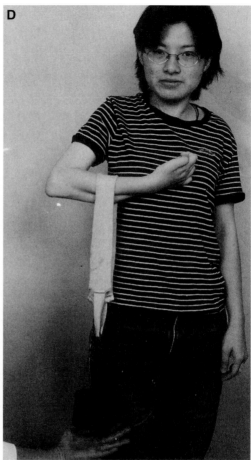

Fig. 2 (*continued*)

spinal accessory nerve transfers are most appropriate for the shoulder, and intercostal nerve transfer is most appropriate for elbow flexion. When available, partial ulnar nerve transfer is best used for elbow flexion. The author prefers to use the contralateral C7 transfer for hand flexors and sensation.

Hypoglossal nerve or deep cervical motor branches are used as adjuvant nerves for the shoulder, when the phrenic nerve is injured, and the diaphragm paralyzed.

7. All the previously described donor nerves can be used to innervate a functioning free muscle for various functions [6,28].

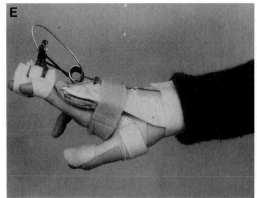

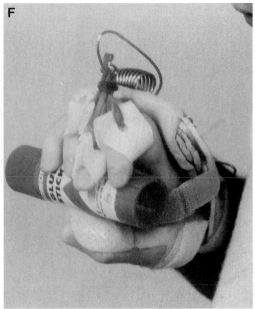

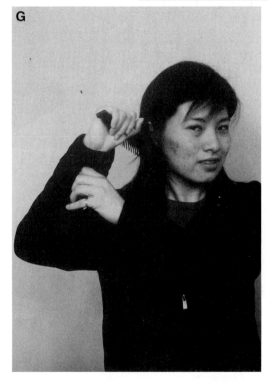

Fig. 2 (*continued*)

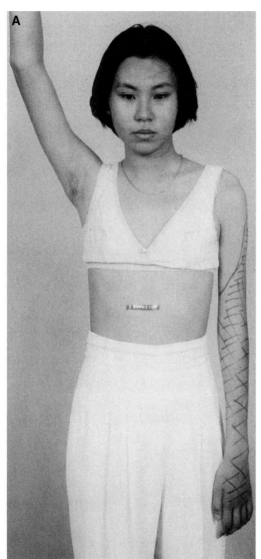
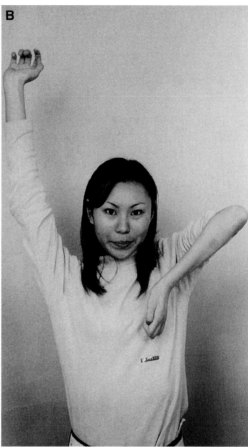

Fig. 3. A 17-year-old girl sustained total root avulsion of the left brachial plexus with complete limb paralysis (*A*). Six years after multiple nerve transfers (performed in one operation), she had regained some function. The reconstruction included the following: spinal accessory nerve transfers to the suprascapular nerve and phrenic nerve to the posterior division of the upper trunk for shoulder function, three intercostal nerve neurotizations of the musculocutaneous nerve for elbow flexion, and contralateral C7 transfer to the median nerve for the hand. (*B–F*) Interphalangeal joint extension was provided by a dynamic splint and improved thumb positioning was provided by an opposition splint.

Reconstructive strategy of nerve transfers: philosophy, experiences, and strategy changes

The anatomy and surgical access of the available donor nerves have been described [8,9,17]. Reconstructive strategies for neurotization procedures have changed over time. The following sections describe the philosophy, experiences, and reconstructive strategy evolution at the author's institution:

Shoulder elevation (or abduction)

The relative priority of active shoulder abduction or adduction depends on an individual surgeon's philosophy. Shoulder adduction provides

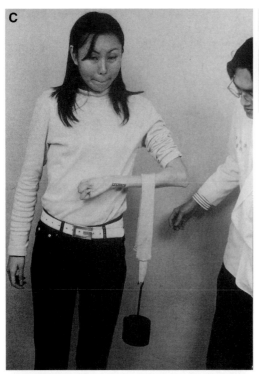

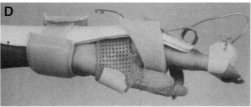

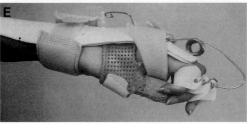

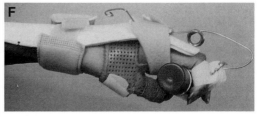

Fig. 3 (*continued*)

an increase in shoulder-to-trunk grasp power, but strong shoulder abduction can provide greater range of motion for the arm and forearm. Shoulder fusion is technically difficult, and the very limited range of shoulder excursion achieved is not appreciated by patients. Therefore, the current author prefers shoulder abduction for reconstruction. Shoulder abduction is a very complex mechanism, requiring synchronous, coupled movements of the scapula and humerus and the coordinated action of at least eight muscles to achieve full abduction of the shoulder. This situation is why neurotization for shoulder abduction in upper plexus avulsion (C5, C6, or C7) will usually have better results than in global or root avulsion when the same is used.

In the author's experience, if supraspinatus, infraspinatus, and deltoid muscles are innervated simultaneously, an average of 60° of shoulder abduction is possible in patients with total root avulsions, and an average of 90° or more is possible in patients with upper root avulsions. Supraspinatus and infraspinatus muscles are innervated by the suprascapular nerve, and deltoid muscle is innervated from the axillary nerve. Axillary nerve reinnervation from spinal accessory or phrenic nerve transfer always requires a long nerve graft (>10 cm). To avoid this situation, the author shifts the spinal accessory nerve or phrenic nerve to the posterior division of the upper trunk, sparing the necessity of a nerve graft, because the axillary nerve arises from the posterior division of the upper trunk. The phrenic nerve is a strong donor nerve. When used to neurotize the C5 root or posterior division of the upper trunk, it can reinnervate the deltoid. At times, triceps and extensor carpi radialis function will be restored at the same time. When both spinal accessory and phrenic nerve are used together, the amount of shoulder abduction obtained is superior to that seen in a single nerve transfer.

Another change in strategy is the author's method of spinal accessory nerve use. Doi et al [6] developed a free-muscle transplantation for extensor digitorum communis (EDC) replacement, which is innervated by the XI nerve (spinal accessory nerve), with impressive results. The current author's experience has been similarly satisfactory. The author now saves the spinal accessory nerve in cases of total root avulsion for a free-muscle transplantation in the late secondary stage. This method not only achieves EDC function but also enhances elbow flexion.

Elbow flexion or extension

In 1992, the author reported using intercostals nerve transfer for musculocutaneous nerve and the success rate was 66% [27]. The success rate (M [muscle strength, scale system M0-M5 based on MRC scale], ≥3) is now ranged from 70% to 90%, with an average of 80%. Three intercostal nerves are still recommended as the donor nerve. The target musculocutaneous nerve is cut close to its lateral cord origin without including the coracobrachialis muscle branch. The distal stump of the musculocutaneous nerve is then moved to the axillary fossa for suture to the intercostal nerves. Five clinical signs of functional recovery appear at different times during the postoperative course. The earliest sign is the biceps squeeze test, in which biceps squeezing induces chest pain. This sign usually appears in the first 3 postoperative months. The second recovery sign is visible biceps contraction, without actual elbow joint movement (M1), during deep inspiration. This sign usually appears 3 to 6 months postoperatively. At this point, induction exercise is then encouraged, including walking or running a minimum of 2 km per day. The third recovery sign is elbow movement with elbow support (gravity eliminated, M2), which usually appears 6 to 12 months post surgery. The fourth recovery sign is elbow flexion against gravity (M3), which appears 12 to 18 months post surgery. Once the muscle strength has reached M3, power can be increased by

resistance exercise. Strength steadily increases at a rate of 0.5 kg every 6 months up to a 3 to 6 kg weightlifting maximum. Intercostal nerves may also be used to innervate a free-muscle transplant for elbow flexion, and remain a good option in chronic cases [28]. The success rate is similar to direct intercostal nerve to musculocutaneous nerve transfers in early cases (ie, ~80%). Intercostal nerve to median nerve transfer is only effective in children with obstetric brachial plexus palsy. These transfers are also not suitable for radial, axillary, or more proximal spinal nerve reinnervation, because this usually ends in a poor result.

Oberlin [17] used a partial ulnar nerve transfer to the musculocutaneous nerve and obtained impressive results with subclinical deficits of ulnar nerve. Since 2002, the current author has used this method preferentially for elbow flexion in patients with upper trunk lesions (C7–T1 intact). In this setting, the Oberlin method is technically easier, recovery is faster, complications are fewer, and the result is superior or equal to that in intercostal nerve transfer.

Finger flexion (or extension)

The restoration of function below the elbow in the subtotal (C7–T1 root avulsions accompanied by rupture or avulsion of C5 or C6) and total root avulsion (C5–T1) is the biggest challenge to brachial plexus surgeons. It is impossible to restore all functions, such as intrinsic muscle functions in the hand and supination/pronation in the forearm. Interphalangeal joint (proximal and distal) extension and thumb internal rotation can be helped by the static or dynamic splint (see Figs. 2 and 3). Forearm pronation can be helped by shoulder abduction, and forearm supination helped by rerouting biceps muscle when the biceps muscle strength is ≥M4. An unstable wrist can be fixed by wrist arthrodesis. Therefore, the main restoration is focused on finger flexion (function of flexor digitorum sublimus or profundus), extension (function of EDC), and sensation. The neurotization of the median nerve, either from ipsilateral C5 or C6 or from contralateral C7 to obtain finger flexion and sensation remains the only possible surgical procedure.

Double-functioning free-muscle transplantation technique in a two-stage procedure [6] is the other method to achieve finger extension and flexion. Nerve neurotization is preferred over double free-muscle transplantation. The nerve neurotization procedure is a reconstruction from "proximal to distal" (ie, from shoulder to elbow to hand in reconstruction priority), which is a more physiologic and logical procedure. Double free-muscle transplantation is a reconstruction from distal to proximal (ie, hand to elbow to shoulder). The latter procedure needs additional sensory neurotization for hand sensation. The hand sensation is obtained by sensory nerve neurotization, such as intercostal nerves or supraclavicular nerve transfer to the median nerve.

Strategy of surgical management for different root injuries

Single-root avulsion

C5 single-root avulsion

Shoulder abduction can be achieved by the following types of transfers: one donor nerve transfer, such as spinal accessory nerve transfer to the suprascapular nerve; two donor nerve transfer, such as spinal accessory nerve and phrenic nerve combined transfers; or three donor nerve transfer, such as a combined phrenic, spinal accessory nerve, and cervical motor branch nerve transfer to the distal C5 spinal nerve. The more donor nerves used, the higher the success rate.

C6 single-root avulsion

A single C6 avulsion is usually associated with C5 rupture, allowing the C5 fibers to be transferred to the anterior division of the upper trunk for elbow flexion. The phrenic nerve is then transferred to the posterior division of the upper trunk, and the spinal accessory nerve is transferred to the suprascapular nerve for shoulder abduction.

C7 single-root avulsion

In this clinical situation, C5 and C6 or the upper trunk itself is ruptured. The repair of the upper trunk is sufficient for shoulder function. There is no need for C7 reinnervation.

C8 single-root avulsion

A single C8 avulsion is usually associated with C5 through C7 rupture or avulsion. The transfer of the C6 or C5 nerve fibers to the C8 nerve with free nerve grafts, accompanied by other extraplexal neurotization procedures for C6 or C5, is recommended.

Two-root avulsions

C5 and C6 root avulsion

Phrenic and cervical motor branch nerves are transferred to the posterior division of the upper trunk, and the spinal accessory nerve moved to the suprascapular nerve for shoulder abduction. Three intercostal nerves are then transferred to the musculocutaneous nerve for elbow flexion.

C6 and C7 root avulsion

This type of avulsion is usually associated with C5 rupture. The C5 nerve fibers are transferred to the distal C6 or anterior division of the upper trunk for elbow flexion. Combined phrenic, spinal accessory, and cervical motor branch nerves are moved to the distal C5 for shoulder abduction.

C8 and T1 root avulsions

These avulsions are usually associated with C5 through C7 ruptures. C5 is transferred for shoulder abduction. The C6 transfer is to the C8 or median nerve for hand function. Intercostal nerves are moved to the musculocutaneous nerve for elbow flexion. The ipsilateral C7 nerve fibers, if available, are usually connected to the distal C7 only, because its transfer for critical function provides unreliable results in the author's experience.

Three-root avulsions

C5, C6, and C7 root avulsion

Phrenic, cervical motor branch, and spinal accessory nerves are transferred for shoulder abduction. Intercostal nerves are used for elbow flexion.

C7, C8, and T1 root avulsion

When C5 and C6 are ruptured rather than avulsed, C5 is used for shoulder abduction; C6 to C8 or median nerve is used for hand function. Intercostal nerves are transferred to the musculocutaneous nerve for elbow flexion.

Four-root avulsions

C6 through T1 four-root avulsion

The C5 root alone is ruptured and usable. Two situations may be encountered: If the C5 stump is healthy, then C5 is transferred to the median nerve for hand function, and phrenic and cervical motor branch nerves are used for shoulder abduction. Intercostal nerves are moved for elbow flexion. The spinal accessory nerve is spared for a later-stage functioning free-muscle transplantation for EDC function. If the C5 stump has questionable health, then C5 is transferred to the posterior division of upper trunk, and the phrenic nerve moved to the suprascaplar nerve for shoulder abduction. Intercostal nerves are used for elbow flexion. The contralateral C7 is transferred to the median nerve with a vascularized ulnar nerve graft for hand function.

All roots avulsed

No plexal roots are available. In this instance, the current author prefers to use the phrenic and cervical motor branches for shoulder abduction. Intercostal nerves are used to provide elbow flexion, and the contralateral C7 transfer is used for hand function. The spinal accessory nerve is spared for a later-stage free-muscle transplantation for EDC replacement.

Summary

The reconstructive strategies for avulsion injuries vary from patient to patient and over time, continue to evolve depending on the surgeon's philosophy, available facilities and therapy, the elapsed time from injury to intervention, the severity of injury, and patient age and motivation. The author's results show that nerve transfer can obtain an average of 60° (range, 20°–180°) of shoulder elevation without shoulder arthrodesis, M3 to M4 muscle strength of elbow flexion, M2 to M4 elbow extension, and M3 finger flexion and sensation. Intrinsic hand function was obtained with help of dynamic splinting for interphalangeal joint extension and arthrodesis of thumb joints as a post for opposition.

References

[1] Narakas A. The surgical management of brachial plexus injuries. In: Daniel RK, Terzis JK, editors. Reconstructive microsurgery. Boston: Little, Brown; 1977. p. 443–68.

[2] Millesi H. Brachial plexus lesions: classification and operative technique. In: Tubiana R, editor. The hand. Philadelphia: WB Saunders; 1988. p. 645–55.

[3] Terzis JK, Vekris MD, Soucacos PN. Outcomes of brachial plexus reconstruction in 204 patients with devastating paralysis. Plast Reconstr Surg 1999; 104:1221–40.

[4] Alnot JY. Traumatic brachial plexus lesions in the adult. Hand Clin 1995;11:623–31.

[5] Chuang DCC. Management of traumatic brachial plexus injuries in adults. Hand Clin 1999;15: 737–55.

[6] Doi K, Sakai K, Kuwata N, et al. Double-muscle technique for reconstruction of prehension after complete avulsion of brachial plexus. J Hand Surg [Am] 1995;20:408.

[7] Jeffert RD. Brachial plexus. In: Green D, editor. Operative hand surgery. 3rd edition. New York: Churchill Livingstone; 1993. p. 1483–516.

[8] Narakas AO. Neurotization in the treatment of brachial plexus injuries. In: Gelberman RH, editor. Operative nerve repair and reconstruction, vol. 2. Philadelphia: JB Lippincott; 1991. p. 1329–58.

[9] Chuang DCC. Neurotization procedures for brachial plexus injuries. Hand Clin 1995;11:633–45.

[10] Millesi H. Nerve grafting. In: Boome RS, editor. The brachial plexus. The hand and upper extremity, vol. 14. New York: Churchill Livingstone; 1997. p. 39–49.

[11] Gu YD. Phrenic nerve transfer for brachial plexus motor neurotization. Microsurgery 1989;10:287–9.

[12] Allieu Y, Privat JM, Bonnel F. Paralysis in root avulsion of the brachial plexus. Neurotization by the spinal accessory nerve. Clin Plast Surg 1984;11: 133–7.

[13] Yeoman PM, Seddon HJ. Brachial plexus injuries: treatment of the flail arm. J Bone Joint Surg [Am] 1961;43:493–500.

[14] Brunelli G, Brunelli F. Use of anterior nerves of cervical plexus to partially neurotize the avulsed brachial plexus. In: Brunelli G, editor. Textbook of microsurgery. Milan, Italy: Masson; 1988. p. 803–7.

[15] Chuang DCC. Brachial plexus neurotization and pedicle muscle transfer. In: Berger RA, editor. Hand surgery. Philadelphia: Lippincott, Williams & Wilkins; 2004. p. 1027–40.

[16] Gu YD, Zhang GM, Chen DS, et al. Seventh cervical nerve root transfer from the contralateral healthy side for treatment of brachial plexus root avulsion. J Hand Surg 1992;17B:518–21.

[17] Oberlin C. Nerve transfer to biceps muscle using a part of ulnar nerve for C5-6 avulsion of the brachial plexus—anatomical studies and report of four cases. J Hand Surg 1994;19A:232–7.

[18] Viterbo F, Trindade JC, Hoshino K, Mazzoni AL. End-to-side neurorrhaphy with removal of the epineurial sheath: an experimental study in rats. Plast Reconstr Surg 1994;94:1038.

[19] Narakas AO. Thoughts on neurotization or nerve transfers in irreparable nerve lesions. Clin Plast Surg 1984;11:153–9.

[20] Narakas AO. Neurotization or nerve transfer in traumatic brachial plexus lesions. In: Tubinan R, editor. The hand. Philadelphia: WB Saunders; 1987. p. 656–83.

[21] Slingluff CL, Terzis JK, Edgerton MT. The quantitative microanatomy of the brachial plexus in man. Reconstructive relevance. In: Terzis JK, editor. Microreconstruction of nerve injuries. Philadelphia: WB Saunders; 1987. p. 285.

[22] Bonnel F. Microscopic anatomy of the adult human brachial plexus: an anatomical and histological basis for microsurgery. Microsurgery 1984;5:107–17.

[23] Bonnel F, Rabischong P. Anatomy and systematization of the brachial plexus in the adult. Anat Clin 1981;2:289–98.

[24] Terzis JK, Papakonstantinou KC. The surgical treatment of brachial plexus injuries in adults. Plast Reconstr Surg 2000;106:1097–122.

[25] Chuang DCC. Contralateral C7 transfer (CC-7T) for avulsion injury of the brachial plexus. Tech Hand Upper Extremity Surg 1999;3(3):185–92.

[26] Chuang DCC, Wei FC. Restoration of shoulder abduction by nerve transfer in avulsed brachial plexus injuries—evaluation of 99 patients with various nerve transfers. Plast Reconstr Surg 1995;96:122–8.

[27] Chuang DCC, Yeh MC, Wei FC. Intercostal nerve transfer of the musculocutaneous nerve in avulsed brachial plexus injuries—evaluation of 66 patients. J Hand Surg 1992;17A:822–8.

[28] Chuang DCC. Functioning free muscle transplantation for brachial plexus injury. Clin Orthop Rel Res 1995;314:104–11.

[29] Richards RR. Operative treatment for irreparable lesions of the brachial plexus. In: Gelberman RH, editor. Operative nerve repair and reconstruction, vol. 2. Philadelphia: JB Lippincott; 1991. p. 1303–27.

[30] Tubiana R. Clinical examination and functional assessment of the upper limb after peripheral nerve lesions. In: Tubiana R, editor. The hand. Philadelphia: WB Saunders; 1988. p. 455.

ELSEVIER
SAUNDERS

Hand Clin 21 (2005) 83–89

HAND
CLINICS

Brachial Plexus Injuries in the Adult. Nerve Transfers: The Siriraj Hospital Experience

Panupan Songcharoen, MD[a],*, Saichol Wongtrakul, MD[a], Robert J. Spinner, MD[b]

[a]Department of Orthopedic Surgery, Faculty of Medicine, Siriraj Hospital, Mahidol University, Bangkok 10700, Thailand
[b]Department of Neurologic Surgery, Orthopedics, and Anatomy, Mayo Clinic/Mayo Foundation, 200 First Street SW, Rochester, MN 55905, USA

Traumatic brachial plexus injuries in adults are commonly caused by motorcycle accidents. Traction may injure the brachial plexus and subclavian vessels as the victim falls off a speeding motorcycle and lands on the hand and shoulder. In many cases, spontaneous improvement does not occur. In examples of postganglionic injury, intraplexal grafting from the C5 and C6 stumps can be performed [1–3]. Commonly, the site of brachial plexus lesion from this mechanism is preganglionic—that is, the proximal anchoring point where the nerve roots leave the spinal cord—which results in a nerve root avulsion. This kind of lesion cannot be treated by conventional nerve repair or nerve grafting [4–7]. Promising work on reimplanting nerves back into the spinal cord has been performed in the laboratory; however, preliminary clinical work shows that this procedure remains at an experimental stage [8–11]. Currently, neurotization remains the best treatment for root avulsions.

Neurotization means reinnervation of a denervated motor or sensory end-organ. Theoretically, there are five types of neurotization, but only neuroneural and neuromuscular neurotization have been used in the treatment of traumatic lesions of the brachial plexus [12–16]. At present, the donor nerves that have been used for neuroneural neurotization of brachial plexus include extraplexal and intraplexal sources. Extraplexal sources include the following: spinal accessory

nerve [17–22], phrenic nerve [22–26], intercostal nerve [13,14,27–29], cervical plexus [12], seventh cervical spinal nerve from the contralateral side [30–32], and hypoglossal nerve [33,34]. Intraplexal sources include the following: ulnar nerve [35–37] or median nerve fascicle [38], long thoracic nerve [39–41], medial pectoral nerve, triceps branch nerve [42], and, recently, ipsilateral C7 nerve root [43]. Results of the most commonly performed nerve transfers for shoulder abduction and elbow flexion are reviewed in a recent meta-analysis [44]. Neurotized free-functioning muscle transfers are being used increasingly as part of a primary or secondary reconstruction to provide various functions, including elbow flexion, wrist extension, and finger extension and flexion [45–47].

Materials and methods

From October 1984 to October 2003, 1449 adult patients with traumatic brachial plexus palsy were treated at Siriraj Hospital (Bangkok, Thailand). There were 1157 nerve transfers performed in these patients to restore the affected limb function.

Functional priority

Restoring elbow flexion has been the main functional priority, followed by shoulder abduction. Hand sensibility and prehension are next considered as part of strategic surgical planning.

Plan of surgical treatment

For the upper arm type of brachial plexus injury with C5,6 or C5,6,7 root avulsions,

* Corresponding author.
E-mail address: sips@mahidol.ac.th
(P. Songcharoen).

shoulder abduction was restored by phrenic to suprascapular neurotization (direct) and elbow flexion was restored by spinal accessory to musculocutaneous neurotization by means of an interpositional sural nerve graft (Fig. 1). Newer techniques for the upper pattern brachial plexus lesion allow the potential for earlier and better recovery. Such an approach could include a fascicular transfer of the ulnar or median nerve to the biceps motor branch or the transfer of a triceps branch to the axillary nerve.

For complete avulsions of C5 through T1 treated before 1 year, the restoration of a hook grip can be attempted with a paradigm of multiple neurotizations, such as the following: a phrenic nerve transfer to the suprascapular nerve, a spinal accessory nerve transfer to the musculocutaneous nerve with an interpositional graft, and a hemicontralateral C7 nerve transfer to the median nerve for wrist and finger flexion and palmar sensation (Fig. 2). Additional techniques can be attempted, such as nerve transfer of the lateral cutaneous nerve to the branch to the extensor carpi radialis brevis. Intercostal nerves can be used to neurotize the triceps and power a free gracilis transfer for finger extension. With adequate recovery, a bone block opponensplasty can be added and static flexion of the metacarpophalangeal joints can be provided.

In late cases of complete avulsion of C5 through T1, the authors have abandoned this algorithm of multiple nerve transfers because of

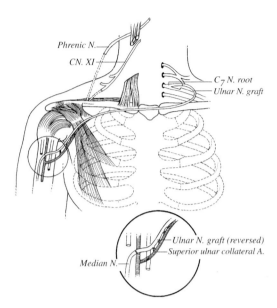

Fig. 2. For complete avulsion injury, a strategy of multiple neurotizations using spinal accessory, phrenic, and contralateral C7 nerves provides a patient with a framework to obtain hook grip. A, artery; CN XI, cranial nerve 11; N, nerve.

poor results. Instead, they have modified it to include a two-stage free-muscle procedure. The first stage consists of free-muscle transfer using spinal accessory nerve neurotization for combined elbow flexion and finger extension. This stage is combined with a hemicontralateral C7 transfer to the median nerve for palmar sensation. A second stage free-muscle transfer could be performed later using the anterior interosseous nerve or intercostal nerve for finger flexion. If recovery were obtained, a third procedure could be designed to allow opposition of the thumb and static metacarpophalangeal joint flexion.

Results

The fifth to sixth cervical nerve stump

In patients with avulsions of C6 throughT1 or C7 through T1 roots, the extraforminally injured C5 or C6 roots or both can be used as donors for plexo-plexal nerve grafting. The most frequently encountered problem with this method of intraplexal nerve grafting is co-contraction of antagonistic muscles. Another commonly encountered problem of plexo-plexal grafting is the method used to determine whether the root stump is an

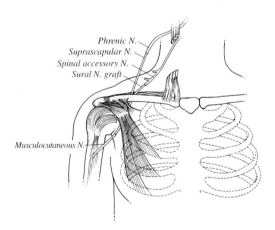

Fig. 1. For upper arm–type avulsion, a reliable neurotization strategy has included phrenic–suprascapular nerve transfer and spinal accessory nerve (with an interpositional nerve graft) to musculocutaneous nerve. N, nerve.

appropriate donor. At present, the use of the microscopic appearance of the proximal stump seems to be the most practical approach to this problem. In the senior author's experience of performing plexo-plexal grafts in 16 patients, 12 patients had gained more than Medical Research Council (MRC) grade 3 motor function after 2 years. Successful recipients included the posterior cord and suprascapular, musculocutaneous, axillary, and median nerves.

Spinal accessory nerve

The spinal accessory nerve (the eleventh cranial nerve) arises from two separate origins: the cranial and the spinal parts. Only the spinal portion of the nerve is used in neurotization of the brachial plexus. This portion of the nerve is predominantly motor in nature. It innervates the sternocleidomastoid and trapezius muscles. The nerve is transected as far distally as possible where the nerve dives deeply to innervate the inferior portion of the trapezius. This technique preserves all of the branches to the sternocleidomastoid and the proximal branches to the trapezius (to minimize the denervation of the trapezius, a muscle that is also innervated in part by the cervical plexus). At this level, the spinal accessory nerve usually contains 1300 to 1600 myelinated nerve fibers.

In the senior author's experience, the percentages of useful motor recovery (MRC grade 3 or better) based on 577 spinal accessory nerve transfers to suprascapular, musculocutaneous, and axillary nerve are 80%, 74%, and 60%, respectively. The spinal accessory nerve can be directly transferred to the suprascapular nerve without using an intermediate nerve graft. Patients with good results from spinal accessory–suprascapular neurotization usually obtain shoulder abduction of 70°, flexion of 60°, and external rotation of 30°. The average recovery time of MRC Grade 3 function was 17.5 months. The musculocutaneous nerve is nearly as good as a recipient. Its main drawbacks are as follows: First, an interpositional nerve graft is necessary. The other drawback is its mixture of both motor and sensory fibers within the same recipient. To prevent the motor fiber loss, a much longer intermediate graft is needed between the spinal accessory nerve and the motor branch to the biceps. Another potential solution is the direct neuromuscular neurotization of the lateral cutaneous nerve of the forearm into the biceps muscle [5]. The best result in the senior

author's series of a spinal accessory–musculocutaneous neurotization allowed a patient to lift a weight of 5 kg to 90° of flexion of elbow and 2 kg to 90° of flexion for 100 times. The spinal accessory–axillary neurotization (also with an interpositional graft) is a moderately good alternative to the spinal accessory–suprascapular neurotization for restoration of shoulder abduction. The patient can obtain 60° of shoulder abduction and 45° of flexion without external rotation. The neurotization of other nerves, including the radial and median nerve, has yielded poor results.

Phrenic nerve

The phrenic nerve originates mainly from the C4 nerve root, with additional branches arising from the C3 and C5 nerve roots. The main trunk of the phrenic nerve is formed at a point midway between the mandible and the clavicle. It runs along the anterior scalene in the neck before entering into the thorax and mediastinum. The phrenic nerve carries efferents to the diaphragm and afferent fibers from the pericardium, pleura, and peritoneum. An accessory phrenic nerve is present in 25% to 38% of patients.

The senior author's experience includes 306 phrenic neurotizations. Of the 151 patients who had a post period operative follow up period of more than 2 years, none had any clinical symptoms or signs of respiratory insufficiency or postoperative respiratory complications. Postoperatively, 27% of the patients had normal diaphragmatic movement, with normal pulmonary function tests, and 73% of the patients had diminished pulmonary function. The vital capacity was reduced by an average of 9.4%. The vital capacity gradually returned to the preoperative level after 6 to 24 months. In the author's experience, the percentage of useful motor recovery (MRC grade 3 or better) after the phrenic nerve was transferred to the suprascapular, musculocutaneous, and axillary nerves was 75%, 60, and 66%, respectively.

The senior author believes that the suprascapular nerve is the best recipient for phrenic neurotization. This procedure can generally be performed without an interpositional nerve graft. Patients with good results obtain 70° of shoulder abduction and 30° of external rotation. The average time to recovery to MRC grade 3 function is approximately 8 months. When the phrenic nerve is harvested in the cervical region and transferred to the axillary nerve and the musculocutaneous nerve, an intermediate nerve graft is needed. Patients with good results from phrenic–axillary neurotization obtain 70° of shoulder abduction and forward flexion. Patients with good results from phrenic–musculocutaneous neurotization can lift a 2-kg weight to 90° of elbow flexion. The involuntary movement of the neurotized biceps gradually changes to a voluntary movement after 2 years. The senior author has no experience with the recently published technique of thoracosopic harvesting of the phrenic nerve as proposed by Xu et al [27]. This endoscopic technique would allow the harvesting of an extended length of phrenic nerve (avoiding the need for an interpositional graft to these target muscles, shortening the time for reinnervation by the end-organ, and potentially improving outcomes).

Before a phrenic nerve transfer is considered, diaphragmatic and pulmonary function must be assessed. The impairment of hemidiaphragmatic movement is an absolute contraindication of phrenic neurotization. In patients who sustain a severe chest injury with multiple rib fractures, the phrenic neurotization should be delayed until the fractures are well healed. Phrenic and intercostal neurotization in the same setting should be avoided. Phrenic neurotization is contraindicated in young infants, because infants born with diaphragmatic paralysis usually have severe respiratory complications. Careful long-term follow-up evaluation is needed to determine any pulmonary sequelae from this technique.

Hemicontralateral C7

In 1986, Gu first transferred the C7 nerve root from the contralateral side to treat a complete brachial plexus avulsion injury. In 1991, Brunelli observed that an isolated avulsion of the C7 nerve root produced only a minimal degree of morbidity in the affected limb. Theoretically, this surgical procedure greatly helps surgeons solve the problem of donor axon inadequacy because the C7 root contains 18,000 to 40,000 fibers. In the current authors' practice, only half of the contralateral C7 is used to minimize the functional deficit of the donor side. This donor contralateral hemi-C7 stump also is a good size match to the vascularized ulnar nerve graft to which it is connected. In general, the authors prefer to target the contralateral C7 to the median nerve but also have performed this technique to the radial or

musculocutaneous nerves. Contralateral C7 neurotization can be performed in patients who have sustained a complete root avulsion brachial plexus injury with concomitant spinal accessory, intercostal, phrenic, and cervical plexus injury. It cannot be performed in patients with bilateral brachial plexus injuries.

The senior author has reported on his operative experience of 111 patients with contralateral C7 neurotizations to the median nerve. Of the patients treated in the primary procedure group who were followed up for more than 3 years, 30% gained a good (M3) motor function and 20% had M2 function. The percentage of protective sensory recovery (sensory grade 2 or more) was 83%. Approximately 50% regained S3 sensory and 33% regained S2 function. The average time to MRC grade S3 motor and a sensory grade 3 recovery was 35 months. Postoperatively, 97% of patients had paresthesias in the index pulp area, median nerve area, or shoulder area; all patients recovered by 7 months (average, 3.75 mo). Three patients had postoperative motor weakness: two involving the triceps (grade 4) and one involving the extensor digitorum communis (grade 2). The triceps weakness recovered in 2 months.

Intercostal nerve

The intercostal nerve contains approximately 3000 to 4000 myelinated fibers, and each intercostal nerve carries a different amount of motor and sensory fibers [48]. The third and fourth intercostal nerves contain a significant amount of motor fibers. The senior author prefers the method of intercostal neurotization as proposed by Tsuyama and Hara [29] and finds it to be the most practical method, giving the best results. Using this technique, the third and fourth intercostal nerves are transferred directly to the musculocutaneous nerve nearest to its motor point without using a nerve graft.

In the senior author's experience, the intercostal nerve transfer to the musculocutaneous nerve restores biceps function in a high percentage of cases. Of 22 intercostal–musculocutaneous neurotizations, 65% of the patients gained a good (MRC grade 3 or better) biceps recovery. The average time to an MRC grade 3 motor recovery is 12 months. The patients with the best recovery could lift a weight of 5 kg to 90° of flexion. During the first 2 years after the operation, biceps function synchronizes with the respiratory cycle. In the third postoperative year, voluntary biceps control is usually attained but involuntary contraction while coughing and sneezing still persists. Sensory recovery in the musculocutaneous nerve area is also obtained. During the first 4 years, sensation is perceived only in the chest. Later, some sensation is also noted in the neurotized area. The results of intercostal nerve transfers to other recipients are generally much poorer.

Cervical plexus

According to Brunelli [6], the cervical plexus has eight branches: four motor and four sensory. The motor branches contain an average of 4090 fibers and the sensory, 3250. The author's experience with three cervical plexus–musculocutaneous neurotization was disappointing. None of the patients recovered MRC grade 3 motor function. The combined use of motor branches of the cervical plexus and the spinal accessory nerve as donors for neurotization must be carefully planned to avoid the risk of denervation of the scapulothoracic muscles. The current authors consider the cervical plexus as a good sensory neurotizer rather than a reliable motor neurotizer.

Fascicles from the ulnar nerve or median nerve of the ipsilateral side

In upper root avulsion brachial plexus injury, the fascicles from the ulnar nerve of the ipsilateral side can be used to neurotize the motor branch to the biceps to restore elbow flexion. The procedure can be done without permanent functional deficit of the donor ulnar nerve. The functional recovery time of biceps is shorter than other neurotization procedures.

The senior author has used this technique for the treatment of upper root avulsion–type brachial plexus injuries in 40 patients. Twenty-four patients had more than 2 years' follow-up evaluation, and 87.5% of the patients regained an M3 or better strength. The elbow flexion power ranged from 1 to 6 kg. The average M3 recovery time was 7.1 months. Postoperatively, six patients (17%) showed clawing of the hand and weakness of grip and pinch strength, which fully recovered by 13 months. Three patients had paresthesias in the ulnar nerve area, which gradually recovered within 3 months.

The main advantage of this procedure is the rapid motor recovery time because the transfer is performed so close to the target muscle (within centimeters of the biceps muscle), without using any interpositional nerve graft. This procedure is especially useful for treatment for patients with upper pattern avulsion injury in whom the elapsed time between injury and operation is more than 6 months. The selection of a fascicle with fibers predominantly to the flexor carpi ulnaris minimizes donor morbidity. The senior author believes that the Oberlin transfer is one of the most reliable neurotization procedures for restoration of elbow flexion, but further study is needed to minimize the functional deficit of the donor nerve.

In 2001, the senior author reported on the use of a fascicle from the ipsilateral median nerve to restore biceps function in upper pattern root avulsion brachial plexus injury. At present, he has used this technique in 15 patients. Ten patients had follow-up evaluation for more than 2 years. Approximately 80% of patients regained an M3 or better biceps strength. The average time for recovery of M3 function was 8 months. Postoperatively, four patients had transient paresthesias in the median nerve distribution. One patient had MRC grade 3 weakness of flexor digitorum profundus and superficialis, flexor pollicis longus, and abductor pollicis brevis with decreased sensation, which gradually improved to MRC grade 4 by 18 months. A fascicle that innervates the flexor carpi radialis muscle is still being sought.

Other nerves (eg, long thoracic, hypoglossal, medial pectoral, thoracodorsal, triceps, ipsilateral C7)

The senior author has limited or no first-hand experience performing the following nerve transfers: long thoracic, hypoglossal, medial pectoral, triceps, and ipsilateral C7.

The long thoracic nerve cannot be used in upper root avulsions because it originates from these roots. Only one or two of the terminal rami can be used to avoid a complete paralysis of the serratus anterior, which leads to a gross dissociation of scapulothoracic motion.

Outcomes following hypoglossal nerve transfer in brachial plexus reconstruction have been disappointing [33,34]. Malessy et al [34] reported the outcomes of hypoglossal nerves transferred to suprascapular and musculocutaneous nerves to treat brachial plexus root avulsion injury. Only 21% of 14 patients had regained MRC grade 3 or better motor recovery. Volitional control was never achieved, and muscle contraction could only be obtained by tongue movement.

For upper pattern brachial plexus injuries, other potential donors exist. Several groups have advocated the use of the medial pectoral nerve or thoracodorsal as transfers in upper pattern avulsion injuries with good success [44]. Recently, Leechavengvongs et al [42] reported excellent results with the long head of the triceps branch transfer to the axillary nerve, achieving shoulder abduction of 124°. Gu et al [43] has used the ipsilateral C7. Reports on the use of end-to-side techniques in brachial plexus reconstruction are also emerging [35].

Summary

A strategy that uses the selective combination of neurotizations can yield a moderate degree of shoulder and elbow control. Even though some wrist and finger movement can occasionally be achieved by the current methods of neurotization, the results in terms of restoration of useful hand function are still far from satisfactory. The use of intraplexal and contralateral plexal neurotization combined with free-functioning muscle transfer and the better understanding of central-peripheral function integration may provide more purposeful hand function in the future.

References

[1] Kline DG, Hudson AR. Nerve injuries: operative results for major nerve injuries, entrapments, and tumors. Philadelphia: WB Saunders; 1995.

[2] Malessy MJA, van Duinen SG, Feirabend HKP, Thomeer RT. Correlation between histopathological findings in C-5 and C-6 stumps and motor recovery following nerve grafting for repair of brachial plexus injury. J Neurosurg 1999;91:636–44.

[3] Seddon H. Nerve grafting. J Bone Joint Surg 1963; 45:447–61.

[4] Azze RJ, Mattar R, Ferreira MC, Starck R, Canedo AC. Extaplexal neurotization of brachial plexus. Microsurgery 1994;15:28–32.

[5] Brandt KE, Mackinnon SE. A technique for maximizing biceps recovery in brachial plexus reconstruction. J Hand Surg [Am] 1993;18:726–33.

[6] Brunelli G. Direct neurotization of severely damaged muscles. J Hand Surg 1982;7:572–9.

[7] Brunelli GA, Brunelli GR. The fourth type of brachial plexus lesion. J Hand Surg [Br] 1991;16:492–4.

[8] Bertelli JA, Ghizoni MF. Brachial plexus avulsion injury repairs with nerve transfers and nerve grafts directly implanted into the spinal cord yield partial recovery of shoulder and elbow movements. Neurosurgery 2003;52:1385–90.

[9] Carlstedt T, Grane P, Hallin RG, Noren G. Return of function after spinal cord implantation of avulsed spinal nerve roots. Lancet 1995;346:1323–5.

[10] Carlstedt T, Anand P, Hallin R, Visra PV, Noren G, Sefferlis T. Spinal nerve root repair and reimplantation of avulsed ventral roots into the spinal cord after brachial plexus injury. J Neurosurgery 2000; 93(Spine 2):237–47.

[11] Fournier HD, Mercier PH, Menei P. Lateral interscalenic multilevel oblique corpectomies to repair ventral root avulsions after brachial plexus injury in humans; anatomical study and first clinical experience. J Neurosurg 2001;95:202–7.

[12] Brunelli G, Monini L. Neurotization of avulsed roots of brachial plexus by means of anterior nerves of cervical plexus. Clin Plast Surg 1984;11:149–52.

[13] Chuang DCC, Yeh MC, Wei FC. Intercostal nerve transfer of the musculocutaeous nerve in avulsed brachial plexus injuries: evaluation of 66 patients. J Hand Surg [Am] 1992;17:822–8.

[14] Dolenc VV. Intercostal neurotization of the peripheral nerves in avulsion plexus injuries. In: Terzis JK, editor. Microreconstruction of nerve injury. Philadelphia: WB Saunders; 1987. p. 425–34.

[15] Harris W, Low VW. On the importance of accurate muscular analysis in lesions of the brachial plexus and the treatment of Erb's palsy and infantile paralysis of the upper extremity by cross-union of nerve roots. BMJ 1903;2:1035–8.

[16] Kawai H, Kawabata H, Masada K, et al. Nerve repairs for traumatic brachial plexus palsy with root avulsion. Clin Orthop 1988;237:75–86.

[17] Allieu Y, Privat JM, Bonnel F. Paralysis in root avulsion of the brachial plexus. Neurotization by spinal accessory nerve. Clin Plast Surg 1984;11:133–6.

[18] Songcharoen P. A preliminary report of 200 brachial plexus injuries treated at Siriraj Hospital. J Asian Orthop Assoc 1990;4:27–30.

[19] Songcharoen P. Brachial plexus surgery: a report of 520 cases. Microsurgery 1995;16:35–9.

[20] Songcharoen P, Chotigavanich C. Brachial plexus injury: a report of 289 neurotizations. J Jpn Orthop Assoc 1994;68:S513.

[21] Songcharoen P, Mahaisavariya B, Chotigavanich C. Spinal accessory neurotization for restoration of elbow flexion in avulsion injuries of the brachial plexus. J Hand Surg 1996;21(A):387–90.

[22] Songcharoen P. Neurotization in the treatment of brachial plexus injury. In: Omer G, Spinner M, Van Beek A, editors. Management of peripheral nerve problems. Philadelphia: WB Saunders; 1998. p. 458–64.

[23] Chuang DC, Lee GW, Hashem F, Wei FC. Restoration of shoulder abduction by nerve transfer in avulsed brachial plexus injury: evaluation of 99 patients with various nerve transfers. Plast Reconstr Surg 1995;96:122–8.

[24] Gu YD, Wu MM, Zhen YL, et al. Phrenic nerve transfer for brachial plexus motor neurotization. Microsurgery 1989;10:287–9.

[25] Sungpet A, Suphachatwong C, Kawinwonggowith V. Restoration of shoulder abduction in brachial plexus injury with phrenic nerve transfer. Austral N Z J Surg 2000;70:783–5.

[26] Xu W-D, Gu Y-D, Xu J-G, Tan LJ. Full-length phrenic nerve transfer by means of video-assisted thoracic surgery in treating brachial plexus avulsion injury. Plast Reconstr Surg 2003;110:104–11.

[27] Nagano A, Ochiai N, Okinaga S. Restoration of elbow flexion in root lesions of brachial plexus injuries. J Hand Surg [Am] 1992;17:815–21.

[28] Nagano A, Tsuyama N, Ochiai N, Hara T, Takahashi M. Direct nerve crossing with the intercostal nerve to treat avulsion injuries of the brachial plexus. J Hand Surg [Am] 1989;14:980–5.

[29] Tsuyama N, Hara T. Intercostal nerve transfer in the treatment of brachial plexus injury or root avulsion type. Excerpta Med 1972;351–3 [International 12th Congress Series 291].

[30] Gu YD, Zhang GM, Chen DS, Yan JG, Cheng XM, Chen L. Seventh cervical nerve root transfer from the contralateral healthy side for treatment of brachial plexus root avulsion. J Hand Surg [Br] 1992;17:518–21.

[31] Gu YD, Chen DS, Zhang GM, et al. Long-term functional results of contralateral C7 transfer. J Reconstr Microsurg 1998;14:57–9.

[32] Songcharoen P, Wongtrakul S, Mahaisavariya B, Spinner RJ. Hemi-contralateral C7 transfer to median nerve in the treatment of root avulsion brachial plexus injury. J Hand Surg 2001;26(A):1058–64.

[33] Ferraresi S, Garozzo D, Ravenni R, et al. Hemihypoglossal nerve transfer in brachial plexus repair: technique and results. Neurosurgery 2002;50:332–5.

[34] Malessy MJA, Hoffman CFE, Thomeer RTWM. Initial report on the limited value of hypoglossal nerve transfer to treat brachial plexus avulsions. J Neurosurg 1999;91:601–4.

[35] Franciosi LF, Modestti C, Mueller SF. Neurotization of the biceps muscle by end-to-side neurorrhaphy between ulnar and musculocutaneous nerves. A series of five cases. Chir Main 1998;17:262–7.

[36] Leechavengvongs S, Witoonchart K, Uerpairojkit C, et al. Nerve transfer to biceps muscle using a part of the ulnar nerve in brachial plexus injury (upper arm type): a report of 32 cases. J Hand Surg 1998;23(A):711–6.

[37] Oberlin C, Beal D, Leechavengvongs S, et al. Nerve transfer to biceps muscle using part of ulnar nerve for C5-C6 avulsion of the brachial plexus: anatomical study and report of four cases. J Hand Surg 1994;19(A):232–7.

[38] Sungpet A, Suphachatwong C, Kawinwonggowit V. One-fascicle median nerve transfer to biceps muscle in C5 and C6 root avulsions of brachial plexus injury. Microsurgery 2003;23:10–3.

[39] Narakas AO. Neurotization in the treatment of brachial plexus injuries. In: Gelberman RH, editor. Operative nerve repair and reconstruction. Philadelphia: JB Lippincott; 1991. p. 1329–58.

[40] Narakas AO. Neurotization or nerve transfer in traumatic brachial plexus lesions. In: Tubiana R, editor. The hand, vol.1. Philadelphia: WB Saunders; 1985. p. 656–83.

[41] Narakas AO. Thoughts on neurotization or nerve transfers in irreparable nerve lesions. Clin Plast Surg 1984;11:153–9.

[42] Leechavengvongs S, Witoonchart K, Uerpairojkit C, et al. Nerve transfer to deltoid muscle using the nerve to the long head of the triceps, part II: a report of 7 cases. J Hand Surg 2003;28(A):633–638.

[43] Gu YD, Cai PQ, Xu F, et al. Clinical application of ipsilateral C7 nerve root transfer for treatment of C5 and C6 avulsion of brachial plexus. Microsurgery 2003;23:105–8.

[44] Merrell GA, Barrie KA, Katz DL, Wolfe SW. Results of nerve transfer techniques for restoration of shoulder and elbow function in the context of a meta-analysis of the English literature. J Hand Surg 2001;26(A):303–14.

[45] Akasaka Y, Hara T, Takahashi M. Restoration of elbow flexion and wrist extension in brachial plexus paralyses by means of free muscle transplantation innervated by intercostal nerve. Ann Chir Main Memb Super 1990;9:341–50.

[46] Chuang DC. Functioning free muscle transplantation for brachial plexus injury. Clin Orthop 1995;314:104–11.

[47] Doi K, Muramatsu K, Hattori Y. Restoration of prehension with the double free muscle technique following complete avulsion of the brachial plexus. Indications and long-term results. J Bone Joint Surg 2000;82(A):652–66.

[48] Freilinger G, Holle J, Sulzbruger SC. Distribution of motor and sensory fibers in the intercostal nerves. Plast Reconstr Surg 1978;62:240–4.

ELSEVIER
SAUNDERS

Hand Clin 21 (2005) 91–102

HAND
CLINICS

Functioning Free-Muscle Transfer for Brachial Plexus Injury

Allen T. Bishop, MD

*Division of Hand Surgery, Department of Orthopedic Surgery, Mayo Clinic, 200 First Street SW,
Rochester, MN 55905, USA*

Traumatic brachial plexus injuries are devastating problems that require prompt referral to centers with expertise in diagnosis, surgical treatment, and subsequent rehabilitation. New microneurosurgical techniques described by others referenced in this article have provided acceptably reliable and stronger innervation of the biceps and shoulder musculature using both nerve grafting and nerve transfer techniques. It must be stressed, however, that these methods are only effective when surgical intervention takes place within 6 to 9 months of injury [1–10].

If reinnervation occurs before 1 year, good muscle function can be restored [11,12]; after 1 year, function will at best be poor. If reinnervation is delayed for 18 to 24 months, irreversible changes in the muscle cells develop, with no hope of return of motor function. Thus, any remedial activity designed to preserve the muscles must be instituted well before 1 year has elapsed.

These methods have not provided reliable restoration of wrist or hand function, however. In many instances, delay in treatment or complete avulsion of the brachial plexus limits the surgeon's reconstructive options. The number of available extraplexal donor nerves is limited,and timing of reconstructive procedures becomes critical. Despite favorable results reported for early nerve grafting and transfer techniques for shoulder and elbow function, reported results of grafting or nerve transfer for hand function have been less favorable [8,13]. Further, attempts at restoring function to long-standing denervated muscle have not been generally successful. This situation has

resulted in the use of free-functioning muscle transfers in conjunction with extraplexal motor nerves to restore elbow function in the setting of brachial plexus avulsions when the time from injury to surgery is more than 9 to 12 months [4,14–19].

Function provided when free muscles are included as part of the patient's management may include not only elbow flexion or extension but also wrist and finger extension and grasp, even in cases of complete plexus avulsion [15,17,20–23]. Thus, current treatment algorithms for brachial plexus injury must generally include not only nerve repair, plexo-plexal grafting, and nerve transfer, but also functioning free microsurgical transfer of muscle to provide patients the most functional recovery possible.

Muscle changes with denervation

Although nerve transection will cause changes to both nerve and muscle, the nerve does not limit functional recovery; however, the muscle rapidly loses the ability to become reinnervated [24]. The biochemical, morphologic, and physiologic changes that occur in muscle fibers following denervation have been well described [25] and include muscle atrophy followed by progressive disorganization of the tissue with time. In human muscle, atrophy results in a 50% reduction of muscle fiber diameter after 2 to 3 months of denervation [26,27]. After 4 months, the atrophic process slows and remains relatively stable for several months.

A decrease in the resting membrane potential is the earliest sign of muscle denervation [28], followed by a dramatic and largely uniform

E-mail address: bishop.allen@mayo.edu

hand.theclinics.com

increase in the sensitivity of the extrajunctional membrane to acetylcholine [29], which occurs after 5 to 10 days. After 10 to 21 days of denervation, spontaneous contractions appear in individual muscle fibers. Fibrillation potentials persist as long as any muscle fiber remains, but are difficult to detect after 1 year [30].

Although denervated muscle responds initially to denervation with an increase of acetylcholine receptors, once the intramuscular nerve terminals disappear and muscle ultrastructure is destroyed, muscle no longer responds to nerve regeneration.

Morphologic and structural changes of denervation include a relative increase in sarcolemmal nuclei [12], followed by fading of visible striations near the end of the first year [31]. Muscle fiber fragmentation [27] and disintegration is complete by 2 years, with eventual replacement by fat cells [31].Thus, the major problem facing brachial plexus surgeons is the many months of nerve regeneration time required before innervation is re-established when treatment is delayed or in distal muscles even with prompt treatment. Given that the rate of axon regeneration varies from 1 to 2.5 mm per day in humans [32], muscles that are 50 cm or more from the lesion site are not reinnervated for 1 year or more [33].

Limited number of nerve transfers

Another reason that functioning free muscles are of use is the generally insufficient number of available proximal nerves to control the multiple functions desirable for shoulder, elbow, wrist, and hand function. Because all extraplexal donor nerves can only be reconnected in proximal locations, distal motor nerves cannot be reliably returned to function (because of late reinnervation).

Free-muscle transfer: the solution?

Given that the rate of nerve regeneration is limited, that function cannot be restored to the shoulder or elbow when treatment is delayed, and that hand function cannot be provided except in a minority of cases with nerve transfer, another solution is needed. In the future, physicians may be able to maintain the morphology and ultrastructure of denervated muscle, place nerve grafts directly into the spinal cord, and greatly increase the rate of axonal regeneration. Because these advances have not yet been made, another solution is required if physicians are to restore

prehensile function. The transfer of a healthy, normal muscle to a paralyzed extremity provides such an opportunity.

Wrist and hand function

When patients are seen and treated promptly after injury, nerve transfers or grafts are used in panplexal injury to restore shoulder and elbow function, as described by Chuang and Songcharoen elsewhere in this issue. Hand function, however, requires restoration of both grasp and release in addition to the positioning functions provided by reinnervated shoulder and elbow muscles. The proximal location of the obturator nerve branch to the gracilis muscle permits proximal (shoulder level) neurovascular connections for rapid reinnervation of nerve transfers. Its length (spanning the entire thigh from pubis to pes anserinus) allows distal tendon connections to hand and wrist motor nerves. Such a muscle, crossing shoulder, elbow, and wrist, has the potential to augment function of more proximal joints as well.

Planning a free-muscle transfer

Selection of donor muscle

As with tendon transfers, free-functioning muscles transferred for a specific purpose should have strength and excursion comparable to the paralyzed muscle or muscles they are replacing and be under volitional control [19]. Other necessary qualities are an adequate blood supply through a single vascular pedicle and a single motor nerve appropriately placed to allow reinnervation by direct nerve transfer. It is also important that the muscle be expendable at its donor site. That is, harvest of the muscle should cause no significant loss of function. For the muscle to work properly, the reconstructive plan should include a means to restore antagonist function by some means as well, if function is to be optimal. Means, such as direct reinnervation, tendon transfer, or tenodesis, or even the use of another free muscle, may make this possible. Although several muscles have been used for functional purposes, the rectus femoris and gracilis muscles are most commonly used [4,14,15,17,18,21,34–37]. Other muscles also have been used for brachial plexus indications, including latissimus dorsi, pectoralis major, and tensor fascia lata [38–42]. The selection of muscle is made by consideration of several parameters, including force-generating capacity, excursion, and a muscle's vascular and nerve anatomy.

Strength

The strength of a muscle is determined in part by its ability to generate force, which is a property of its physiologic cross-sectional area. Cross-sectional area is determined by measurements after sectioning the muscle in a plane perpendicular to its fibers. This process requires anatomic dissection and multiple sections in the case of bipennate muscles. More practically, muscle volume determination provides another good measure of force-generating potential. It is therefore useful to compare the cross-sectional area of common donors with recipient sites. The muscle's points of origin and insertion and distance from the joint center of rotation are also important factors to consider [43]. The most commonly used gracilis muscle and to a lesser extent the latissimus are poorly matched to the biceps based on a comparison of their cross-sectional area to that of the elbow flexors, whereas the rectus femoris provides the best fit for strength but not excursion [43]. Experience shows that both the gracilis and latissimus provide acceptable strength.

The satisfactory results obtained by gracilis transfers for elbow function, reported by many authors, defy expectations based on their anatomic measurements [4,15,34,36,37,44–49]. It seems that any of the commonly used muscles may provide acceptable strength for function, although the exceptional length, proximal neurovascular pedicle, and excellent distal tendon of the gracilis have made it the preferred choice of most authors.

Excursion

Not all muscles have the same amount of excursion, or length of pull, of the distal tendon. Excursion is directly related to muscle fiber length and indirectly affected by fiber orientation relative to the long axis of the muscle. In general, excursion is approximately equal to 40% of resting muscle fiber length [43]. Excursion should ideally equal or exceed normal motion at the recipient site. Strap muscles, in which fibers run parallel to the muscle axis, provide more excursion than pinnate muscles, whose orientation is oblique to the muscle. Other factors, such as fascial connections or postoperative scarring of muscle and tendon, will limit excursion, as will anatomic

considerations after transfer, such as bowstringing across the elbow joint or the need to stabilize or move more than one joint with a single muscle [15]. Excursion requirements for hand function range from approximately 3 cm for wrist flexion or extension to approximately 7 cm for finger flexion. Finger extension is intermediate to these values. In comparison, the mean resting fiber length of the gracilis is 26 cm, the latissimus, 23 to 28 cm, and the rectus femoris, 8 cm [50].

Other muscle factors

Other factors play a role in muscle selection, the most important of which are the quality of the distal and proximal tendons and the vascular and motor nerve anatomy. The vascular anatomy relevant to free-muscle transfer of muscles was described by Mathes and Nahai [51]. According to their classification, muscles with a single vascular pedicle (type I) or those with a dominant vascular pedicle and either multiple minor (type II) or secondary segmental (type V) pedicles may be transferred with the expectation of muscle survival. The most commonly used gracilis is a type II muscle, whereas the rectus femoris is type I and the latissimus dorsi type IV.

Patient requirements for functioning free-muscle transfer

As in any complex procedure, not all patients are good candidates for reconstruction. Patients must be sufficiently motivated to undertake such an operation but also able to take responsibility for the extensive rehabilitation that will be required during the subsequent 2 years. Helping the patient to understand the nature of the procedure and the required perioperative and postoperative care before the procedure is undertaken requires considerable time on the part of the surgical team, but these steps are important if the patient is to participate in his or her care.

Proximal joint stability and balance are also helpful in obtaining a good outcome. In the plexus, shoulder stability is important. A recent study compared the effectiveness of grasp after double free-muscle transfer in patients with no shoulder reconstruction versus those who had either shoulder girdle muscle reinnervation or glenohumeral arthrodesis [52]. The authors concluded that shoulder function is important for achieving prehensile function among patients with complete paralysis of brachial function, when they undergo double free-muscle transfer.

Adequate or reconstructable skin cover and bed for tendon gliding is important for a muscle to function normally. If the muscle is used to both provide soft tissue coverage and function, as is sometimes necessary in massive upper extremity injury associated with brachial plexus injury, the resultant excursion of the muscle may prove insufficient for functional joint range of motion.

There must be an expendable motor nerve in the vicinity of the muscle neurovascular pedicle to provide animation. Extraplexal nerves are usually used, including, most commonly, the spinal accessory nerve and intercostal motor nerves. The evaluation of trapezius function by examination of shoulder shrug, compared with the opposite side, and by electromyography (EMG) is required when its use is planned. Similarly, chest inspiration/expiration radiographs, chest percussion for diaphragmatic excursion, and preoperative pulmonary function tests should be obtained before the phrenic nerve is selected. The intercostal nerves may have been injured in the chest wall injuries commonly associated with plexus trauma. Chest radiograph, EMG, and direct evaluation of intercostal nerves at surgery with nerve stimulation should be used before proceeding with muscle harvest.

The local vasculature must be sufficient to permit successful microvascular repairs. The physician cannot count on physical examination of peripheral pulses to provide sufficient preoperative planning information before free-muscle transfer. To prevent unpleasant surprises, including potential loss of the transfer in the perioperative period, a formal magnetic resonance angiogram or conventional angiographic study is a routine part of the author's preoperative assessment for all patients in whom a functioning free-muscle transfer is planned. The incidence of axillary or subclavian artery avulsion has been reported to be as high as 10% to 25% [53,54], especially in association with first rib and other extremity fractures. At times, the vessel wall of otherwise patent vessels may be thickened, or terminal branches, such as the thoracoacromial trunk, may show substantial injury even when the major vascular supply to the extremity is intact. In such circumstances, the physician must be prepared to find alternative solutions to a planned anastomosis.

Uses of free-muscle transfer

For brachial plexus indications, free muscles are most commonly used in two situations: (1) Free muscles are used for restoration of elbow flexion alone in late-presenting patients with no other alternatives. (2) In patients seen within 6 months of injury, free-muscle transfers are often performed in combination with other nerve grafts and/or nerve transfers. Either single or double muscle transfers are used in this setting. Such reconstructions require a through understanding of all possible reconstructive options and the functional priorities for motor function. In general, elbow flexion carries the highest priority, followed by shoulder stability or motion, grasp function, hand sensibility, and intrinsic function. The availability of multiple nerves for transfer may permit more reliable or more functional results when combined with free muscles used to provide animation for grasp and release function of the hand.

Single gracilis transfer

Free-muscle transfers provide reliable elbow flexion when treatment delay prevents direct graft or biceps neurotization and proximal muscle strength is insufficient to allow tendon transfers [4,15,34,36,37,44–49]. At times, a single transfer may also prove useful for other functions, including shoulder abduction, elbow extension, or finger flexion [15]. In the author's experience, 79% of the gracilis free-functioning muscle transfers for elbow flexion alone (single transfer; Fig. 1) achieved at least M4 elbow flexion strength [15].

Double gracilis transfer

Doi et al [17,21,23,55] have described a method to provide shoulder stability and function combined with active elbow flexion and extension, hand sensibility, and rudimentary hand grasp and release function in patients with four or five root avulsions. The double free-muscle transfer takes advantage of the length of the gracilis muscle and proximal location of its neurovascular pedicle to promote rapid reinnervation of the muscle while allowing for distal joint function. A direct neurotization of the spinal accessory nerve to a gracilis muscle fixed to the clavicle can produce elbow flexion and finger or wrist extension (Fig. 2), whereas the second transfer, secured to the second rib and neurotized to intercostal motor nerves, creates finger flexion (Fig. 3). The creative use of additional intercostal nerves for triceps function and sensory neurotization of the hand allows

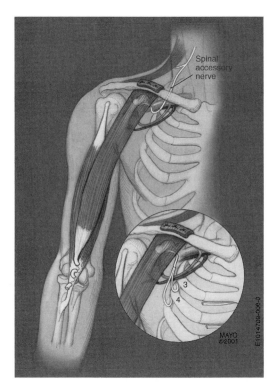

Fig. 1. The gracilis functioning free-muscle transfer for restoration of elbow flexion. The gracilis is fixed to the clavicle proximally and distally to the biceps tendon. Motor innervation is provided either by the spinal accessory or the third and fourth intercostal motor nerves. Vascular connections are made with the thoracoacromial trunk vessels. (Courtesy of Mayo Foundation and Research, Rochester, MN; with permission.)

independent elbow flexion/extension and hand grasp/release if all components of the procedure are successful (Fig. 4).

Surgical technique (general)

The surgical transfer of a functioning free-muscle transfer is a lengthy procedure, and careful preparation of the patient is important. Adequate padding and positioning to protect bony prominences and provide adequate exposure of donor and recipient sites are critical. The maintenance of body core temperature facilitates peripheral tissue perfusion. The use of fluid warmers, control of ambient temperature, coverage of exposed skin, and use of warming devices should begin as the patient enters the operating room and continue as needed throughout the procedure.

Initial dissection is performed at the recipient site, generally before any dissection of the probable donor muscle is performed. If the soft tissues and skin are in good condition, the initial assessment of the recipient site should determine that a mechanically sound site exists to which the muscle origin may be attached and to ensure a distal insertion will also be possible, generally to the tendon of insertion providing the desired motion.

Verification that recipient site vessels and motor nerves are undamaged is the final major determinant. The current author and others at his institution prefer to use the thoracoacromial trunk for free-muscle vascular anastomoses for elbow flexion or combined elbow flexion and wrist/finger extension, as described by Doi et al [21]. The thoracodorsal vessels are used when the free muscle is transferred for finger flexion. The spinal accessory or intercostal motor nerves provide acceptable nerve function, and the phrenic nerve remains an alternative choice when, as is usually the case, no plexal nerves are available. Staged reconstruction with contralateral C7 also has been described, but only preliminary results have been reported [56]. The author has no experience with this method.

Once nerve and vascular connections are dissected and their adequacy verified, muscle harvest is begun. It is important to minimize muscle ischemic time by careful preparation of the recipient site vessels, including the prevention or correction of vasospasm with topical vasodilators and the verification of adequate outflow before the muscle blood supply is interrupted for harvest. The microscope and vascular clamps should be in place, and the muscle origin and insertion points exposed and prepared for immediate repair before muscle transfer.

The dissection of the recipient nerve should maximize its length, and the probable required length of donor motor nerve should be determined to ensure that no interposition graft will be necessary. At the donor site, every attempt is made to maximize vessel and nerve length, because extra tissue is easily excised but inadequate vessel or nerve cannot be easily corrected. The author also prefers to harvest all muscles, including a cutaneous flap, for monitoring purposes.

Gracilis harvest

The gracilis is a superficial muscle that lies on the medial aspect of the thigh. A branch of the obturator nerve enters the muscle obliquely just cephalad to the major vascular pedicle, at a point

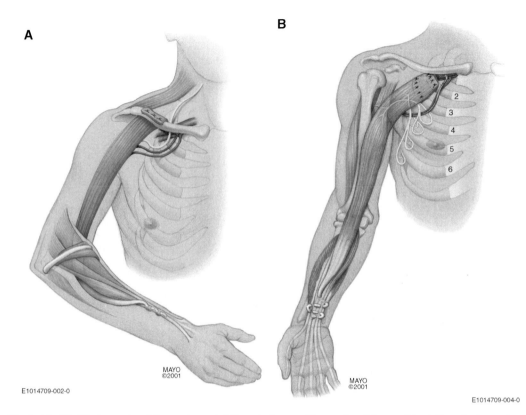

Fig. 2. Modified Doi stage 1 and 2 procedures. (*A*) Stage 1: free gracilis transferred for combined elbow flexion and wrist extension. Usually combined with neurotization of shoulder girdle musculature as well (not shown). (*B*) Stage 2: a second functioning free gracilis tranfer is performed for finger flexion using two intercostal motor nerves. Additional nerve transfers are performed for triceps neurotization and hand sensibility (see Fig. 3). (Courtesy of Mayo Foundation and Research, Rochester, MN; with permission.)

6 to 12 cm from its origin. The dominant arterial supply is provided by a branch from the profunda femoris artery 8 to 12 cm from the muscular origin and is approximately 4 to 6 cm long. Maximal dissection of the obturator nerve can obtain 10 cm or more of length, greatly facilitating nerve transfers without interpositional grafting at the recipient site. The muscle is released from the pubic symphysis proximally and from its tendinous insertion at the pes anserinus distally. The gracilis is routinely transferred with a skin paddle for postoperative flap monitoring [19].

Once transferred, the tendon of origin is expeditiously repaired. The author uses suture anchors preplaced in the clavicle to quickly attach the gracilis for elbow flexion, for example. The muscle is tunneled and provisionally placed in its final position, but without final tension adjustment before vascular repairs. The author then proceeds quickly to complete the vascular anastomoses and restore perfusion, generally with

1 hour or less of ischemia time. Meticulous neurorrhaphy is then performed with epineural sutures and fibrin glue as close to the muscle as possible to minimize reinnervation time.

Appropriate muscle tension is important for a good result, and can most easily be based on restoration of the original muscle resting length using superficial sutures placed at measured intervals along the length of the muscle before dissection, as originally described by Manktelow [19,57] and Manktelow et al [58]. Appropriate tenodesis effect should be noted for the desired transfer because proximal joint motion either tenses or relaxes the muscle.

Single gracilis transfer method

In the author's experience, transfer of a single gracilis for elbow flexion, generally performed in late-presenting patients with the limited goal of elbow flexion alone, is a reliable procedure when

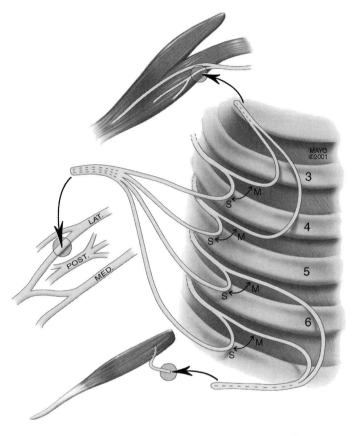

Fig. 3. Motor and sensory neurotizations performed in the second stage of the double free-muscle procedure. The triceps is reinnervated with the third and fourth intercostal motor nerves, whereas the fifth and sixth intercostals are used for the free gracilis (finger flexion). Sensory portions of each intercostal nerve are transferred to the lateral cord contribution to the median nerve for hand sensation. (Courtesy of Mayo Foundation and Research, Rochester, MN; with permission.)

two to three intercostal motor nerves or the spinal accessory nerve is used for motor neurotization. In the cases involving intercostal neurotization, the intercostal motor nerves were exposed through either an inframammary or a parasternal incision, the latter used early in the author's experience, or when a simultaneous pectoralis major flexorplasty was performed [15]. Subperiosteal mobilization of the third and fourth ribs exposes the intercostal muscle and avoids injury to the pleura. Blunt dissection in the cephalad portion of each intercostal muscle identified the intercostal motor nerve, confirmed by use of a nerve stimulator. Intercostal nerves 3 and 4 were primarily used as donor nerves based on their close proximity to the harvested gracilis neurovascular pedicle. The intercostal nerves were dissected distally to the point at which muscle

contraction ceased (generally near the costal chondral cartilage junction) and proximally to the anterior axillary line.

When the spinal accessory nerve was used, it was identified on the deep anterior surface of the trapezius muscle, confirmed by use of a nerve stimulator. The most proximal motor branch to the trapezius was identified and protected to preserve muscle function. The remainder of the motor branch was mobilized for neurotization, sacrificing other trapezial motor branches as necessary to facilitate mobilization and nerve transposition beneath the clavicle. The brachial artery (8 patients), thoracoacromial trunk (4 patients), axillary artery (2 patients), and lateral pectoral artery (1 patient) were used for the arterial anastomosis, and their venae comitantes or the cephalic vein was selected for venous anastomosis.

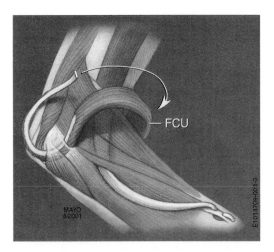

Fig. 4. Creation of a flexor carpi ulnaris (FCU) pulley at the antecubital fossa prevents development of postoperative bowstringing of the stage 1 free-muscle transfer. (Courtesy of Mayo Foundation and Research, Rochester, MN; with permission.)

In patients seen within 3 to 6 months of injury, surgical exploration of the brachial plexus was performed and confirmation of root avulsion obtained by intraoperative somatosensory evoked potentials (SEPs) before selecting free-muscle transfer. In long-standing paralysis, no plexus exploration was undertaken. The gracilis muscle was dissected and the recipient site prepared to receive the transfer before its vascular pedicle was divided. Once freed from the leg, it was brought immediately to the arm and positioned within the recipient site, in most cases for elbow flexion. In such cases, it is desirable to position the gracilis muscle as close to the donor motor nerve as possible to minimize reinnervation time and avoid the use of an intercalated nerve graft. When the spinal accessory nerve is to be used, this step is accomplished by fixing the gracilis proximally by placement beneath the clavicle and wrapping the muscle around the cephalad and anterior clavicle surface. The gracilis is then sutured into place through multiple clavicle drill holes. The dissection of the spinal accessory nerve as distally as possible generally permits its passage beneath the clavicle in close proximity to the base of the gracilis neurovascular pedicle. The muscle is tunneled subcutaneously to a separate antecubital incision. End-to-end or end-to-side arterial repairs are acceptable. When the thoracoacromial trunk is used (the author's preference for elbow flexion transfers), direct end-to-end arterial repair is most appropriate, followed by venous anastomosis.

The distal tendon was secured to the biceps tendon by means of a Pulvertaft weave following completion of the vessel anastomoses and neurorrhaphy (see Fig. 1). Tensioning of the transferred muscle was performed with the arm held in 30° of flexion with the muscle at its normal resting length.

Double gracilis transfer method

The double free-muscle transfer was originally described by Doi [59]. The author and others at his institution have performed nine such transfers, using a slightly modified technique [15]. The technique for reconstruction of the upper extremity following complete brachial plexus avulsion consists of two surgical procedures, each using a gracilis muscle transfer. The first stage consists of surgical exploration of the brachial plexus with SEP monitoring. At present, shoulder motor reconstruction is routinely performed, either using an available C5 nerve root, phrenic nerve, or contralateral hemi-C7 transfer [13]. The first gracilis free-muscle transfer restores elbow flexion and finger or wrist extension. The gracilis is secured to the clavicle proximally as previously described. The distal tendon is tunneled beneath the mobile wad just proximal to the elbow and sutured to the extensor carpi radialis brevis tendon in the proximal portion of the forearm. Tensioning of the muscle transfer is such that full elbow flexion is permitted with a 30° flexion contracture and simultaneous passive finger or wrist extension, but allowing full wrist flexion with the elbow flexed. The first gracilis transfer is neurotized to the spinal accessory nerve, and the vascular pedicle is anastomosed to the thoracoacromial trunk (see Fig. 2).

The second gracilis transfer restores finger flexion. Proximally, the gracilis is secured to the second rib through multiple drill holes. Distally, a second incision is made in the forearm and the flexor digitorum profundus and flexor pollicis longus tendons are identified and sutured together in a position that creates key pinch and grasp with traction. The distal tendon is tunneled from the arm to the forearm beneath the pronator teres to create a pulley effect. The tendon is woven into the previously prepared flexor digitorum profundus and flexor pollicis longus tendons using a Pulvertaft weave. The graft is tensioned to allow the fingers to extend with elbow flexion and to permit the fingers and thumb to close with elbow extension. The second gracilis transfer is neurotized by two intercostal motor nerves, and the vascular pedicle is anastomosed to the thoracodorsal artery and vein (see Fig. 2).

In addition to the second gracilis transfer, the second stage of the double free-muscle transfer requires neurotization of two intercostal motor nerves to the motor branch of the triceps brachii muscle (see Fig. 3). The restoration of elbow extension allows the ability to better control distal joint function provided by the functioning free muscles crossing the elbow by allowing its active stabilization. In addition, sensory neurotization of the lateral portion of the median nerve with sensory intercostal nerves is performed to restore protective hand sensibility (see Fig. 3).

Aftercare

Postoperatively, the patients are monitored for 48 hours in an ICU, which permits frequent assessment of the muscle by skin color, turgor and capillary refill, and Doppler examination of myocutaneous perforators. Adequate fluids are important to maintain peripheral perfusion, and the ambient temperature is maintained at 80°F during this period. Passive range of motion of uninvolved joints and edema control are begun immediately.

Thereafter, patients are progressively mobilized, and they are usually dismissed from the hospital on the fifth postoperative day. The shoulder and all joints involved in the muscle transfer are immobilized for 3 weeks, then gentle passive range-of-motion exercise is begun. Subsequent rehabilitation is discussed in another section of this article.

Results: single free-muscle transfer

Many authors have reported excellent results when a single gracilis muscle is transferred for restoration of elbow flexion [4,15,34,36,37,44–49]. In the author's experience, functional results were obtained in 79% of all such cases [15]. The use of intercostal and spinal accessory nerves provided equivalent results. In 2 of the 17 such cases, no muscle function was recovered despite demonstrable muscle survival.

Results: double free-muscle transfer

Using a double free-muscle transfer, Doi et al [17] was able to restore excellent to good elbow flexion in 96% of his patients. In addition, 65% achieved more than 30° of total active motion of the fingers with the second muscle transfer.

At the author's institution, he and his colleagues have slightly modified the double free-muscle transfer, as originally described by Doi. In stage 1, the gracilis muscle is secured to wrist extensors as opposed to finger extensors, because the author and colleagues believe this helps promote finger flexion through a tenodesis effect. In addition, the author and others have recently altered the route of the first gracilis muscle transfer to create a more effective pulley at the elbow using the flexor carpi ulnaris muscle. When the brachioradialis muscle was used to create a pulley, as originally described by Doi, the author and colleagues have routinely encountered bowstringing of the first gracilis muscle transfer at the elbow. To create a more effective pulley, they now detach the distal portion of the flexor carpi ulnaris and create a pulley at the level of the proximal forearm (see Fig. 4). They believe this will improve muscle excursion and strengthen wrist extension.

In performing the double free-muscle transfers, the author and colleagues have been unable to consistently restore prehension, although in general, some active flexion was achieved. Although they routinely observed both survival and active contraction of the second muscle transfer, they believe that, in most cases with poor results, a tenolysis would have improved active motion. Scarring of the wrist and finger tendons is a major postoperative problem encountered with free-functioning muscle transfers. It may be that modification of surgical techniques, such as the use of silicone wraps, may be necessary to promote tendon gliding. Doi et al [17] also noted improved active finger flexion after performing a tenolysis in patients in whom there was poor active finger flexion despite strong contraction of the transferred muscle. In their study, 9 of 26 patients who underwent a gracilis transfer for combined restoration of elbow range of motion and prehension had significantly improved finger range of motion following tenolysis of the muscle transfer.

Of nine patients in the current author's series, eight had follow-up evaluation for 1 year or more. Transfer for combined elbow flexion and wrist extension compared with elbow flexion alone lowered the overall results for elbow flexion strength to a strength of 63% of M4 or greater, compared with 79% in single function transfers. Grasp function was less reliable, with five of eight patients having at least some finger motion (average, 30° total active motion [TAM]). Only two patients in the study underwent a secondary tenolysis procedure, largely because many of these patients were unavailable for follow-up evaluation. Patient inability or unwillingness to return at regular intervals for examination, therapy, and subsequent surgery, and poor compliance with postoperative therapy, at times made appropriate aftercare difficult or impossible. It was the author's clear impression that many of these young men had socioeconomic factors adversely affecting their ability to fully cooperate with the rehabilitation program. Although all patients were encouraged to participate in postoperative rehabilitation, most of the patients had less than 1 year of rehabilitation. This noncompliance with postoperative rehabilitation may explain why the author and colleagues were unable to duplicate the results seen in many of the Asian studies.

In the Mayo study, the transfer of a gracilis for combined elbow flexion and wrist or finger extension diminished slightly the number of patients who achieved M4 strength [15]. Although it is possible to achieve good to excellent outcomes in terms of muscle grades with the simultaneous reconstruction of two functions by one free-muscle transfer, more reliable results are obtained with the transfer of a single muscle for a single function. Doi et al [52,60] has emphasized the importance of both shoulder stability and triceps recovery to improve the results of free-muscle transfers, which, of necessity, span the shoulder, elbow, or both to produce distal joint function.

Summary

Functioning free-muscle transfers are now an important, even essential, tool in the current management of patients with brachial plexus injury. They are indicated for the restoration of elbow flexion in patients who delay presentation (those seen after 6 to 9 mo). Double free-muscle transfers provide the possibility of simple grasp function when combined with nerve transfers or grafts for restoration of shoulder motion, hand sensation, and triceps function.

References

[1] Allieu Y, Cenac P. Neurotization via the spinal accessory nerve in complete paralysis due to multiple avulsion injuries of the brachial plexus. Clin Orthop 1988;237:67–74.

[2] Chuang DC. Neurotization procedures for brachial plexus injuries. Hand Clin 1995;11:633–45.

[3] Chuang DC, Lee GW, Hashen F, Wei FC. Restoration of shoulder abduction by nerve transfer in avulsion brachial plexus injury: evaluation of 99 patients with various nerve transfers. Plast Reconstr Surg 1995;96:122–8.

[4] Krakauer JD, Wood MB. Intercostal nerve transfer for brachial plexopathy. J Hand Surg [Am] 1994; 19(5):829–35.

[5] Leechavengvongs S, Witoonchart K, Uerpairojkit C, Thuvasethakul P, Ketmalasiri W. Nerve transfer to biceps muscle using a part of the ulnar nerve in brachial plexus injury (upper arm type): a report of 32 cases. J Hand Surg [Am] 1998;23(4):711–6.

[6] Merrell GA, Barrie KA, Katz DL, Wolfe SW. Results of nerve transfer techniques for restoration of shoulder and elbow function in the context of a meta-analysis of the English literature. J Hand Surg [Am] 2001;26(2):303–14.

[7] Mikami Y, Nagano A, Ochiai N, Yamamoto S. Results of nerve grafting for injuries of the axillary and suprascapular nerves. J Bone Joint Surg [Br] 1997;79:527–31.

[8] Narakas AO, Hentz VR. Neurotization in brachial plexus injuries. Indication and results. Clin Orthop Rel Res 1988;237:43–56.

[9] Ruch DS, Friedman A, Nunley JA. The restoration of elbow flexion with intercostal nerve transfers. Clin Orthop Rel Res 1995;314:95–103.

[10] Songcharoen P, Mahaisavariya B, Chotigavanich C. Spinal accessory neurotization for restoration of elbow flexion in avulsion injuries of the brachial plexus. J Hand Surg [Am] 1996;21(3):387–90.

[11] Stewart DM, Sola OM, Martin AW. Hypertrophy as a response to denervation in skeletal muscle. J Physiol [Lond] 1972;76:146–67.

[12] Sunderland S, Ray LJ. Denervation changes in mammalian striated muscle. J Neurol Neurosurg Psychiatry 1950;13:159–77.

[13] Songcharoen P, Wongtrakul S, Mahaisavariya B, Spinner RJ. Hemi-contralateral C7 transfer to median nerve in the treatment of root avulsion brachial plexus injury. J Hand Surg [Am] 2001;26(6): 1058–64.

[14] Akasaka Y, Hara T, Takahashi M. Free muscle transplantation combined with intercostal nerve crossing for reconstruction of elbow flexion and wrist extension in brachial plexus injuries. Microsurgery 1991;12(5):346–51.

[15] Barrie KA, Steinmann SP, Shin AY, Spinner RJ, Bishop AT. Gracilis free muscle transfer for restoration of function after complete brachial plexus avulsion. Neurosurg Focus 2004;16(5):15.

[16] Berger A, Flory P-J, Schaller E. Muscle transfers in brachial plexus lesions. J Reconstr Microsurg 1990; 6:113–6.

[17] Doi K, Muramatsu K, Hattori Y, et al. Restoration of prehension with the double free muscle technique

following complete avulsion of the brachial plexus. Indications and long-term results. J Bone Joint Surg [Am] 2000;82(5):652–66.

[18] Doi K, Sakai K, Kuwata N, Ihara K, Kawai S. Reconstruction of finger and elbow function after complete avulsion of the brachial plexus. J Hand Surg [Am] 1991;16(5):796–803.

[19] Manktelow RT. Functioning muscle transplantation to the upper limb. Clin Plast Surg 1984;11(1): 59–63.

[20] Doi K, Hattori Y, Kuwata N, et al. Free muscle transfer can restore hand function after injuries of the lower brachial plexus. J Bone Joint Surg [Br] 1998;80(1):117–20.

[21] Doi K, Kuwata N, Muramatsu K, Hottori Y, Kawai S. Double muscle transfer for upper extremity reconstruction following complete avulsion of the brachial plexus. Hand Clin 1999;15(4):757–67.

[22] Doi K, Sakai K, Fuchigami Y, Kawai S. Reconstruction of irreparable brachial plexus injuries with reinnervated free-muscle transfer. Case report. J Neurosurg 1996;85(1):174–7.

[23] Doi K, Sakai K, Kuwata N, Ihara K, Kawai S. Double free-muscle transfer to restore prehension following complete brachial plexus avulsion. J Hand Surg [Am] 1995;20(3):408–14.

[24] Finkelstein DI, Dooley PC, Luff AR. Recovery of muscle after different periods of denervation and treatments. Muscle Nerve 1993;16(7):769–77.

[25] Sunderland S. Nerves and nerve injuries. 2nd edition. New York: Churchill Livingstone; 1978.

[26] Adams RD. In: Diseases in muscle: a study in pathology. 3rd edition. New York: Harper & Row; 1975. p. 112–30.

[27] Aird RBN, et al. The pathology of human striated muscle following denervation. J Neurosurg 1935; 10:216–24.

[28] Thesleff S. Physiological effects of denervation of muscle. Ann N Y Acad Sci 1974;228:89–103.

[29] Lømo T, Westgaard RH. Further studies on the control of ACh sensitivity by muscle activity in the rat. J Physiol [Lond] 1975;252:603–26.

[30] Barwick DD. In: Walton J, editor. Clinical electromyography: disorders of voluntary muscle. 4th edition. New York: Churchill Livingstone; 1981. p. 952–75.

[31] Bowden REM, Gutmann E. Denervation and reinnervation of human voluntary muscle. Brain 1944; 67:273–313.

[32] Sunderland S. Rate of regeneration in human peripheral nerves. Arch Neurol Psychiatry 1947;58: 251–95.

[33] Eberstein A, Pachter BR. The effect of electrical stimulation on reinnervation of rat muscle: contractile properties and endplate morphometry. Brain Res 1986;384(2):304–10.

[34] Akasaka Y, Hara T, Takahashi M. Restoration of elbow flexion and wrist extension in brachial plexus paralyses by means of free muscle transplantation

innervated by intercostal nerve. Ann Chir Main Memb Super 1990;9(5):341–50.

[35] Chuang DC. Functioning free muscle transplantation for brachial plexus injury. Clin Orthop Rel Res 1995;314:104–11.

[36] Chung DC, Carver N, Wei FC. Results of functioning free muscle transplantation for elbow flexion. J Hand Surg [Am] 1996;21(6):1071–7.

[37] Sungpet A, Suphachatwong C, Kawinwonggowit V. Transfer of one fascicle of ulnar nerve to functioning free gracilis muscle transplantation for elbow flexion. Aust N Z J Surg 2003;73(3):133–5.

[38] Favero KJ, Wood MB, Meland NB. Transfer of innervated latissimus dorsi free musculocutaneous flap for the restoration of finger flexion. J Hand Surg [Am] 1993;18(3):535–40.

[39] Hovnanian AP. Latissimus dorsi transplantation for loss of flexion or extension at the elbow. Ann Surg 1956;143:494.

[40] Ihara K, Shigetomi M, Kawai S, Doi K, Yamamoto M. Functioning muscle transplantation after wide excision of sarcomas in the extremity. Clin Orthop Rel Res 1999;358:140–8.

[41] Lu L, Gong X, Liu Z, Wang D, Zhang Z. Diagnosis and operative treatment of radiation-induced brachial plexopathy. Chin J Traumatol 2002;5(6): 329–32.

[42] Takami H, Takahashi S, Ando M. Latissimus dorsi transplantation to restore elbow flexion to the paralysed limb. J Hand Surg [Br] 1984;9(1):61–3.

[43] Doi K, Hattori Y, Tan SH, Dhawan V. Basic science behind functioning free muscle transplantation. Clin Plast Surg 2002;29(4):483–95, v–vi.

[44] Baliarsing AS, Doi K, Hattori Y. Bilateral elbow flexion reconstruction with functioning free muscle transfer for obstetric brachial plexus palsy. J Hand Surg [Br] 2002;27(5):484–6.

[45] Doi K, Sakai K, Ihara K, Abe Y, Kawai S, Kurafuji Y. Reinnervated free muscle transplantation for extremity reconstruction. Plast Reconstr Surg 1993; 91(5):872–83.

[46] Friedman AH, Nunley JA II, Goldner RD, Oakes WJ, Goldner JL, Urbaniak JR. Nerve transposition for the restoration of elbow flexion following brachial plexus avulsion injuries. J Neurosurg 1990; 72(1):59–64.

[47] Hattori Y, Doi K, Ohi R, Fukushima S, Baliarsing AS. Clinical application of intraoperative measurement of choline acetyltransferase activity during functioning free muscle transfer. J Hand Surg [Am] 2001;26(4):645–8.

[48] Ikuta Y, Yoshioka K, Tsuge K. Free muscle graft as applied to brachial plexus injury—case report and experimental study. Ann Acad Med Singapore 1979;8(4):454–8.

[49] Oberlin C. Brachial plexus palsy in adults with radicular lesions, general concepts, diagnostic approach and results [in French]. Chir Main 2003; 22(6):273–84.

[50] Krimmer H, Hahn P, Lanz U. Free gracilis muscle transplantation for hand reconstruction. Clin Orthop Rel Res 1995;314:13–8.

[51] Mathes SJ, Nahai F. Classification of the vascular anatomy of muscles: experimental and clinical correlation. Plast Reconstr Surg 1981;67(2): 177–87.

[52] Doi K, Hattori Y, Ikeda K, Dhawan V. Significance of shoulder function in the reconstruction of prehension with double free-muscle transfer after complete paralysis of the brachial plexus. Plast Reconstr Surg 2003;112(6):1596–603.

[53] Gupta A, Jamshidi M, Rubin JR. Traumatic first rib fracture: is angiography necessary? A review of 730 cases. Cardiovasc Surg 1997;5(1):48–53.

[54] Sturm JT, Perry JF Jr. Brachial plexus injuries from blunt trauma—a harbinger of vascular and thoracic injury. Ann Emerg Med 1987;16(4):404–6.

[55] Doi K. New reconstructive procedure for brachial plexus injury. Clin Plast Surg 1997;24(1):75–85.

[56] Chuang DC, Wei FC, Noordhoff MS. Cross-chest C7 nerve grafting followed by free muscle transplantations for the treatment of total avulsed brachial plexus injuries: a preliminary report. Plast Reconstr Surg 1993;92(4):717–25 [discussion: 726–7].

[57] Manktelow RT. Functioning muscle transplantation. In: Manktelow RT, editor. Microvascular reconstruction: anatomy, applications and surgical techniques. New York: Springer Verlag; 1986. p. 151–64.

[58] Manktelow RT, Zuker RM, McKee NH. Functioning free muscle transplantation. J Hand Surg [Am] 1984;9A:32–9.

[59] Doi K. New reconstructive procedure for brachial plexus injury. Clin Plast Surg 1997;24(1):75–85.

[60] Doi K, Shigetomi M, Kaneko K, et al. Significance of elbow extension in reconstruction of prehension with reinnervated free-muscle transfer following complete brachial plexus avulsion. Plast Reconstr Surg 1997;100:364–72.

ELSEVIER
SAUNDERS

Hand Clin 21 (2005) 103–108

HAND
CLINICS

Pre-/Postoperative Therapy for Adult Plexus Injury

Denise Kinlaw, PT, CHT

Department of Physical Medicine and Rehabilitation, Mayo Clinic, Rochester, MN 55901, USA

The rehabilitation of patients who have sustained brachial plexus injuries is essential. Therapy is performed to maintain and increase range of motion (ROM), retard the rate of muscle atrophy, and re-educate the muscles once the reconstructive surgeries have been completed and reinnervation is verified.

The common interventions for all patients with brachial plexus lesions include the following:

1. Slings and splinting
2. Passive ROM (PROM)
3. Massage for edema control and scar management
4. Electrical stimulation
5. Neuromuscular re-education, including electrical stimulation and biofeedback
6. Active, assistive ROM, including use of gravity-minimized positions, powder boards, and skate boards
7. Active ROM
8. Strengthening
9. Sensory re-education

Most of these interventions are used pre- and postoperatively.

Preoperative care

Patients who have an upper trunk or complete brachial plexus lesion often require support to prevent or minimize the inferior glenohumeral subluxation, which results from paralysis of the deltoid, supraspinatus, and infraspinatus muscles. A universal sling, envelope sling, or hemisling may be used for this purpose (Fig. 1). Maintaining normal capsular integrity is important to improve glenohumeral motion once shoulder girdle muscular function recovers. In addition, patients feel more secure when using the sling, because it minimizes the discomfort they often report at the shoulder joint and prevents uncontrolled positional motion of the paralyzed limb. The sling should be adjusted so that the head of the humerus is held in a normal or slightly elevated position in the glenoid. For patients who have incisions in the region of the neck and upper shoulder, the straps of the universal sling lying across that area may be uncomfortable and require modification. Alternatively, some patients prefer taping of the shoulder for the same purpose.

The paralysis of wrist extensors causes a passive, flexed, resting stance of the wrist. It is therefore frequently useful to use a splint to maintain the wrist in 10° to 20° of extension. Either prefabricated or custom splints are satisfactory. The splint may, over time, cause an extension resting posture, which is helpful if digit flexion function remains or recovers. In the initial postinjury period, PROM exercises are done to maintain upper extremity joint mobility. The therapist must be aware of the possible future surgical interventions to ensure an optimum amount of motion is maintained to allow the greatest functional potential. Even in complete avulsion injuries, digit mobility should be aggressively maintained, because grasp function remains a potential goal in some surgical algorithms. Patients are taught to do self-ROM exercises for the best results.

Some surgeons [1,2] recommend electrical stimulation to specific muscles before neurotization surgeries, tendon transfers, or free-muscle transfers. Electrical stimulation for denervated muscles must be performed using direct-current stimulation (Fig. 2). Neuromuscular stimulators with short pulse durations are not effective in the case of injury to lower motor neurons with resultant Wallerian degeneration. Denervated muscles must be stimulated with a unit that is capable of producing direct current with "infinite"

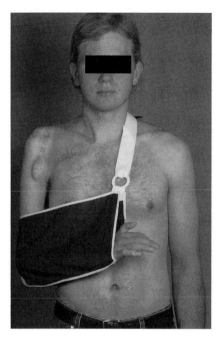

Fig. 1. A universal sling, envelope sling, or hemisling may be used. (Courtesy of Mayo Foundation and Research, Rochester, MN; with permission.)

duration (≥300 ms), because denervated muscle responds to a stimulus differently than normal muscle. The terms used to describe motor response include *rheobase* (the smallest amplitude of current flowing for an infinite duration that produces a minimal but perceptible response) and *chronaxie* (the shortest stimulus time at twice the rheobase that will produce a minimal perceptible response).

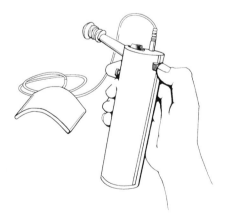

Fig. 2. An example of a stimulation unit designed for home use. (Courtesy of Mayo Foundation and Research, Rochester, MN; with permission.)

Denervated muscle has a chronaxie longer than 20 to 30 milliseconds, most often closer to 100 milliseconds, whereas that of normally innervated muscle is less than 1 millisecond [3].

Immediate postoperative care

After surgery, sufficient time has to be allowed for the nerve and muscle transfers to heal before therapy is begun. The patient is immobilized to allow time for healing to take place in the tissues involved in the surgery. Most commonly, the patient's shoulder girdle is immobilized in a shoulder immobilizer for 3 weeks or more, and a cast or splint is used to protect more distal nerve or tendon connections for 3 to 6 weeks at the surgeon's discretion.

Depending on the lesion and the surgical reconstruction, PROM is indicated as soon as permitted by the surgical team to maintain motion as much as possible. PROM is not to be confused with passive stretching. It is defined as motion within the unrestricted range of a joint [5], whereas stretching implies going beyond this range. Thus, motion of the hand and wrist may be permissible immediately post surgery if no functioning free-muscle or tendon transfers have been performed, whereas the shoulder arc of motion may be more or less permanently restricted to a safe range if intercostal nerves were transferred into the arm. Generalization is not possible because of the wide range of reconstructions performed in modern brachial plexus surgery. A close working relationship between the therapist and physician is therefore required. PROM exercises may be done 4 to 6 times a day or more (Fig. 3). At each exercise session, 10 to 20 repetitions or more may be performed, taking care to stay within the restrictions dictated by the surgeon. Depending on the lesion, certain joints may be allowed to develop contractures to maximize function. This situation may be desired in complete brachial plexopathies. When free gracilis transfers are done, elbow flexion contractures of approximately 30° are desirable to give the patient a better angle of pull so that flexion will be easier to initiate. Wrist extension contractures may allow for better grasp following free-muscle transfer for wrist or finger extension [1].

Edema control and scar management are incorporated into the plan of care. Examples of edema control include decongestive massage, compression sleeves or garments, and elevation as possible. Scar management is included for patients

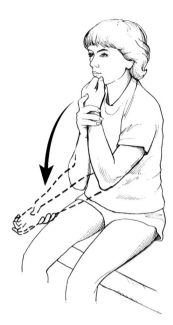

Fig. 3. PROM exercises may be done 4 to 6 times a day or more. (Courtesy of Mayo Foundation and Research, Rochester, MN; with permission.)

who have problems with excessive scarring and adhesions. Scar massage is done to keep the scar mobile. Elastomer pads, gel sheeting, or other materials may be used to help to soften and flatten the scars.

Electrical stimulation is begun 3 to 6 weeks after surgery, which allows time for the nerve transfers to heal with considerably less danger of rupture. Because these are cases of reinnervation, the muscle may not respond to currents that are produced by neuromuscular stimulators. As mentioned previously, a direct-current (galvanic) stimulator is needed. Electrodes are placed to stimulate the muscle directly. If a unit is available that has the ability to vary the pulse duration, use a current duration that is longer than the chronaxie of the muscle. Some units that are available clinically allow for the establishment of rheobase, chronaxie, and a strength-duration (intensity-time) curve [4]. As the muscle reinnervates, the chronaxie slowly decreases. The time at which muscle recovery begins is thus detectable by changes in the stimulation parameters. The time at which recovery begins depends on the length of axonal regeneration required, among other factors. The current author has found that when the chronaxie decreases to 20 milliseconds or shorter, voluntary contractions of the muscle begin [3,4].

If changes in measured chronaxie can be observed and recorded, reinnervation can be surmised, even before a formal electromyographic (EMG) evaluation provides confirmation. The contraction elicited using the direct-current stimulator will be a twitch type, often a slow and "wormlike" twitch initially, becoming brisker as the muscle reinnervates.

To decrease the frequency of supervised therapy, the patient may do electrical stimulation with a portable home unit. The patient may perform two to six stimulation sessions a day. At each session, the patient is instructed to stimulate for 30 to 60 moderately strong contractions. The contractions must be visible. If the patient experiences sensation and has difficulty tolerating the stimulation, the current may be decreased, but there must be a visible contraction. The skin in the insensate limb must be inspected after each session to assess skin breakdown at the electrode sites. If there is a tendency for skin breakdown, vary the electrode placement frequently. The home stimulation unit may be set up for monopolar or bipolar technique, to be determined by the therapist at one of the supervised sessions. An example of one such unit designed for home use is shown in Fig. 2. The unit has a trigger-type on-off switch. There is an extension from the barrel that houses the active electrode. The dispersive electrode is placed on the patient and secured with a rubber strap. The patient and therapist work together to find the best stimulation points. As mentioned previously, it is important to choose alternate sites for stimulation to avoid skin breakdown, given the high number of repetitive stimulations recommended.

Re-education of muscle

In the rehabilitation of recovering function, it is important to have a thorough understanding of the surgical reconstruction, particularly when nerve transfers from intra- or extraplexal sources have been done. The therapist must also have a good working knowledge of functional anatomy, especially regarding the specific motor innervation of commonly transferred nerves, if the patient is to be successful in his or her rehabilitation efforts.

The re-education technique [6] used depends on the type of surgery performed. Common extraplexal sources include the spinal accessory and intercostal nerves, and phrenic and contralateral C7 nerve roots. The most common intraplexal nerve transfer is the use of a portion of the ulnar nerve to restore elbow flexion in high plexus lesions.

The re-education of extraplexal nerve transfers begins when voluntary motor unit potentials are seen on EMG or visible contraction is observed. The patient will usually easily produce successful contraction by replicating the function of the nerve in question. For example, muscles that were neurotized by the intercostals or the phrenic nerve can be activated using breathing techniques. These techniques may include deep breathing, pursed lip breathing, coughing, yawning, or the Valsalva maneuver. For the muscles or transfers that are neurotized with the spinal accessory nerve, elevation of the scapula (shoulder shrug) is used for the re-education process. For the contralateral C7, mirroring motions of muscles that have C7 in their distribution may help to activate the muscles. Most commonly, grasp with the opposite hand will elicit a response in the opposite limb. Functional contraction is often not seen in this instance until 2 to 3 years after the surgery. In the Oberlin technique, fascicles from the ulnar nerve, most commonly those that produce flexor carpi ulnaris activation, are used to restore elbow flexion. Re-education that emphasizes elbow flexion combined with wrist flexion and ulnar deviation will likely be successful, although the use of other ulnar nerve functions, such as finger abduction or adduction, may also be of use. For all recovering muscles, short sessions of re-education are necessary at first to avoid hyperventilation and fatigue. The re-education process makes use of various methods to first obtain and then strengthen the recovering muscles. These methods include biofeedback methods, which include the use of visual or tactile clues, gravity-eliminated exercises, and progressive strengthening techniques.

Biofeedback

When active muscle contractions appear, biofeedback may be used to help the patient key in on the muscle contraction and increase his or her ability to fire the muscle. Again, to decrease the number of supervised sessions, there are portable biofeedback units that the patient may use at home (Fig. 4). In later stages of re-education, biofeedback may also be in the form of visual and palpatory monitoring of the transferred or re-neurotized muscle. The patient's opposite hand or a mirror may also be used to monitor the quality

of the contraction of the transfer once motor control has returned [6].

Other re-education techniques may be used if biofeedback machines are not available. The techniques may include the use of neuromuscular re-education [6] and neuromuscular electrical stimulation. The purpose of neuromuscular electrical stimulation is to give the patient the visualization and sensation of the contraction. The current amplitude of the evoked contraction is strong at first to give the patient the sense of the muscle contracting. The current amplitude is slowly decreased to see if the patient can continue the contraction voluntarily. As the patient gains in the strength of the voluntary contraction, the strength of the stimulus is decreased [7].

Gravity-eliminated exercise

The initial re-education training is in the gravity-eliminated or gravity-reduced positions (Fig. 5). The goal is to be able to attain as much range as possible in the gravity-eliminated position. When maximum available ROM is gained, light weights may be added in the gravity-eliminated position. Trials of antigravity positioning should be done

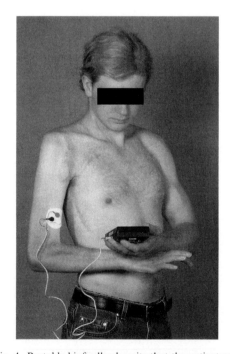

Fig. 4. Portable biofeedback units that the patient may use at home are helpful in the re-education process. (Courtesy of Mayo Foundation and Research, Rochester, MN; with permission.)

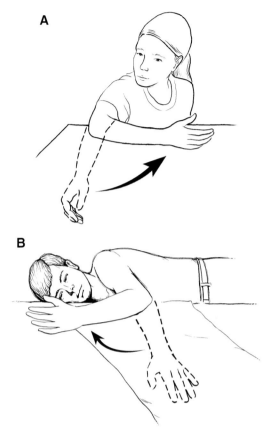

Fig. 5. Positions that may be used for gravity-eliminated exercises include (*A*) sitting (if shoulder abduction is permissible) and (*B*) lying on one's side. (Courtesy of Mayo Foundation and Research, Rochester, MN; with permission.)

periodically to see if there is sufficient strength gain to move in the antigravity position.

Strengthening

As the muscle gains strength, working against gravity will be possible. As re-education advances, biofeedback is a valuable tool, because it allows the patient to monitor improvement in the contraction of the muscle.

When the patient gains antigravity strength, weights may be added to help with strength gains. As the strengthening begins, the weights must be light. It is recommended that the starting weight be about 0.1 to 0.25 kg. The gravity-eliminated position allows the patient to have some success with the weights before progressing to the antigravity positions. The therapist should not hesitate to use isometric, concentric, or eccentric contractions. If the patient is highly motivated, he or she may tend to overdo exercise with the weights. The patient may experience some postexercise soreness when the muscles are overworked.

The strength gains are slow. The therapist is a cheerleader of sorts for the patient, and he or she should encourage the patients often. When possible, it is recommended that the patient be seen every day for the first 2 to 3 months and then every other day. Close supervision will lead to the best results. Even the most highly motivated patients can lose motivation over such a long period of rehabilitation.

Pain management

One of the most difficult areas to deal with is nerve pain. Some patients experience little or no pain and others find the pain to be at times unbearable. In most such cases, evaluation by a specialist in a pain clinic is important. Uncontrolled pain may make it difficult for the patient to use the involved extremity in a functional manner.

Sensory re-education

Perhaps the most difficult aspect of rehabilitation is the sensory re-education. In cases of complete avulsion, the limb is insensate below the shoulder. Surgical reconstruction of sensation may be part of the patient's surgical plan, most often using intercostal sensory, contralateral C7, or cervical plexus branches. The slow process of nerve regeneration from the supraclavicular area to the hand dictates that little or no improvement can be expected for at least 2 years. Patients must be cautioned regarding the possibility of pressure sores, and injury from sharp objects, heat, and cold. Routine inspection of skin is important. Once some perception of sensation is present, there will be a role for sensory re-education. Testing with Semmes-Weinstein monofilaments will help to determine if the patient is ready for sensory re-education. In general, a value of 4.31 is required before such therapy is worthwhile [8].

References

[1] Doi K, Sakai K, Kuwata N, Ihara K, Kawai S. Double free-muscle transfer to restore prehension following complete brachial plexus avulsion. J Hand Surg Am 1995;20(5):408–14.

[2] Terzis JK, Papakonstantinou KC. The surgical treatment of brachial plexus injuries in adults. Plast Reconstr Surg 2000;106(5):1097–124.

[3] Spielholz N. Electrical stimulation of denervated muscle. In: Nelson R, Hayes KW, Currier DP, editors. Clinical electrotherapy. Norwalk (CT): Appleton & Lange; 1999. p. 411–46.

[4] Hayes K. Electrophysiologic measurement. In: Hayes KW, editor. Manual for physical agents. Norwalk (CT): Appleton & Lange; 1993. p. 139–47.

[5] Kisner C, Colby L. Therapeutic exercise, foundations and techniques. 4th edition. Philadelphia: FA Davis; 2001.

[6] Kottke F. Therapeutic exercise to develop neuromuscular coordination. In: Kottke FJ, Lehmann JF, editors. Krusen's handbook of physical medicine and rehabilitation. Philadelphia: WB Saunders; 1990. p. 452–79.

[7] Baker L. Clinical uses of neuromuscular electrical stimulation. In: Nelson R, Hayes KW, Currier DP, editors. Clinical electrotherapy. Norwalk (CT): Appleton & Lange; 1999. p. 355–410.

[8] Hunter J, Mackin E, Callahan A. Sensibility testing with Semmes-Weinstein Monofilaments. In: Hunter J, Mackin E, Callahan A, editors. Rehabilitation of the hand and upper extremity. Philadelphia: Mosby; 2002. p. 194–213.

ELSEVIER
SAUNDERS

Hand Clin 21 (2005) 109–118

HAND
CLINICS

Repair of Avulsed Ventral Nerve Roots by Direct Ventral Intraspinal Implantation after Brachial Plexus Injury

Henri D. Fournier, MD, PhD[a,b,*], Philippe Mercier, MD[a,b], Philippe Menei, MD, PhD[a]

[a]Service de Neurochirurgie, Centre Hospitalier Universitaire, 4 Rue Larrey, 49033 Angers, Cedex 9, France
[b]Laboratoire d'Anatomie, Université d'Angers, Rue Haute de Reculée, 49100 Angers, France

Nerve root avulsion involving the cervical medulla is a common consequence of traumatic traction of the brachial plexus and can cause dramatic damage, including complete paralysis of the upper limb. The prognosis for such lesions—which tend to affect young adults who are the most likely to be involved in road accidents—is poor. This type of avulsion is considered to be a problem of the central nervous system (CNS), and therefore irreparable, by most specialists, even those with extensive experience in plexal surgery. Avulsion is a complication in 70% of cases of severe traction of the brachial plexus [1], and it can contribute to a permanent severance of the cervical cord from peripheral effector muscles. This dissociation leads to the disappearance of motor neurons in the anterior horn of the spinal cord gray matter and is responsible for causalgia associated with interruption of afferent nerve signals (deafferentation pain) [2].

Current surgical modalities are based on neurotization (ie, nerve transfer) and are purely palliative, aiming to stimulate reinnervation of the muscles that depend on the myotomes compromised by avulsion. The muscles of the shoulder and the brachial biceps are the main targets. The most common procedures involve the following: installing a connection between the accessory nerve (XI) or an intercostal nerve and the suprascapular nerve, homolateral or contralateral transfer of the C7 root to the musculocutaneous or median nerve, and fascicular transfer of the ulnar nerve to the brachial biceps nerve (the Oberlin operation) [3–5]. These procedures are based on knowledge and experience accumulated over many years, and they afford improvement in flexion and extension of the elbow. These techniques therefore aim at specific outcomes.

In France, in 2001, an extensive review of the efficacy of these conventional surgical modalities was conducted under the auspices of the Agence Nationale d'Accréditation et d'Evaluation en Santé (ANAES). ANAES is a public administrative establishment with the dual purpose of defining current knowledge about preventive strategies and the diagnosis and treatment of disease and fostering improvement in the quality and safety of care provision, both in public hospitals and in the private sector. For this review, a group of experts conducted a critical and exhaustive analysis of the international literature to evaluate the efficacy of the various surgical options with reference to the method used and the clinical picture and to analyze their safety and the incidence of associated complications. In the process, the evidence presented in each of the relevant articles was attributed a scientifically based level of reliability. The ultimate question addressed by the experts was whether the specific operation should be kept on the list of procedures to be reimbursed by the social security system. The result of this analysis was that, from the evidence, outcomes of surgical approaches to traumatic lesions of the brachial plexus in general

* Corresponding author. Service de Neurochirurgie, Centre Hospitalier Universitaire, 4 Rue Larrey, 49033 Angers, Cedex 9, France.

E-mail address: hdfournier@chu-angers.fr (H.D. Fournier).

hand.theclinics.com

are poor. In a formal consensus position concerning these procedures, however, the experts nevertheless concluded that, given the seriousness of this type of lesion coupled with the absence of any alternative surgical options, continued reimbursement is justified.

Although these conclusions may discourage specialists of the brachial plexus, especially the lack of any positive evidence in the literature indicating that these procedures are of value, they are nonetheless true, and the status of these surgical interventions vis-à-vis reimbursement is delicate.

At a time of progress in the neurosciences, trying to find alternative or complementary solutions to this problem is becoming a priority—and an urgent one.

This is then an ideal moment for research into spinal repair of nerve root avulsion, to work toward developing ways of reducing the lesions in a more global fashion. Without representing a completely alternative option, such an approach could one day be added to the therapeutic arsenal and significantly improve outcomes.

Prior research

In the 1980s, several researchers working with animal models showed that implantation of a peripheral nerve graft into the spinal cord can induce regeneration of spinal motor neurons, which grow a matter of centimeters across the graft [6–11]. From such results, extensive work was performed to investigate the efficacy of implanting peripheral nerve grafts in the cervical cord. This work shed much light on the subject. Six weeks after nerve root avulsion, the death of motor neurons in the anterior horn leaves only 40% of the original neuron population. Direct reimplantation or the implantation of a peripheral graft increases the percentage of residual motor neurons after 6 weeks to 80%, and this process is associated with the regeneration of axons and the restoration of function. Peripheral nerve graft transplantation seems therefore to promote axon regrowth. The main reason for this is that the graft provides a component that is essential for peripheral nerve function, the Schwann cell. It has been shown that the Schwann cell does not die after peripheral transection of the axon, but rather it goes on producing numerous neurotrophic factors and synthesizes certain components of the extracellular matrix, notably laminin (which modulates the neuritic response). It also produces various cell adhesion molecules that stimulate axon regrowth [12–23].

Encouraged by these results, Carlstedt [26] was the first to experiment with reimplantation in humans. Furthermore, intradural exploration of the damaged plexus was first described as early as 1911 [24], and the first attempt to reimplant an avulsed nerve root back into the medulla was reported in 1979 [25]. This work was not followed up until Carlstedt et al [26] published his first case history in 1995. More recently, he and others have published the largest clinical series of patients treated with reimplantation techniques [27]. This study describes 10 patients who had suffered major damage to the brachial plexus. All were operated on with a simple hemilaminectomy by means of a posterior approach, 10 days to 9 months after the injury. A sural nerve graft was implanted into the white matter of the lateral cord after incision to a depth of 1 to 2 mm. The first electromyographic signs of reconnection with the target were detected 9 to 12 months after the operation. In eight patients, the muscle was contracting within 1 year (Medical Research Council [MRC] grade 1/5). In five of these patients, the contraction remained ineffective but three patients had recovered some function (MRC grades 3 to 5) within 3 to 4 years of reimplantation. All three of these patients had been operated on relatively early (between the 10th and the 28th day after the injury). Function was recovered in the biceps, triceps, and deltoid muscles but not in the muscles of the hand. Simultaneous contraction of opposing muscles inhibited movement in some patients. The effect on pain remains uncertain, and in two patients, the procedure was associated with Brown-Séquard's syndrome. In their conclusions, the authors emphasized the importance of intervening as early as possible for a satisfactory long-term outcome.

Thus, the success of this type of procedure is limited, and the procedure itself remains controversial. Nevertheless, these preliminary results are promising and warrant further work. Because of the results obtained in animals, certain constructive extrapolations can be made. The surgical approach used to gain access to the cord to implant the graft may not be the ideal choice in that it fails to afford access to the anterior horn. Moreover, it does not seem to provide access to the infraclavicular brachial plexus, and the site of implantation in the white matter of the lateral cord, which is dictated by this approach, is probably not ideal. A new surgical approach is therefore needed. It is possible that concomitant treatment with the appropriate neurotrophic factors might be able to promote axon regrowth in the white matter.

Ideas such as these led the current authors to focus on this approach, which opens compelling possibilities.

Description of the authors' work

Aims

The current authors hoped to show that reimplantation can work in humans if it is performed correctly, and that it can restore function, even in patients with avulsion of multiple nerve roots controlling several different groups of muscles. The authors also wanted to show that this technique, which restores communication from the spinal cord to the periphery, can diminish or abolish deafferentation pain.

Anatomic basis of the posterior approach to the brachial plexus for repairing avulsed spinal nerve roots

The authors' first step was to understand the work of Carlstedt to account for its relative failure [28]. They therefore focused on the anatomy of the brachial plexus, notably that of the medullary reimplantation compartment and the posterior relationships of the plexus. They undertook this step before examining and treating their first three patients. This early work allowed the authors to adapt the posterior subscapular approach (described many years ago) to the imperatives of reimplantation and, at the same time, define its limitations and sketch out an anatomic explanation for the mediocrity of Carlstedt's results.

The main problem in reimplanting nerve roots is how to expose the whole of the proximal brachial plexus from the intradural rootlets right up to where the branches divide, and do so with a single surgical approach. This step is essential for accurate evaluation of the extent of the damage and for global repair. Avulsion may be associated with damage to the supraclavicular brachial plexus (and, in a few cases, infraclavicular damage, although this is rare). Because the conventional anterior approach to the brachial plexus does not afford access to the intradural compartment, the posterior subscapular approach, as used by Kline et al [29], seemed to represent the only way of evaluating and repairing extensive proximal lesions with the avulsion of multiple nerve roots at different levels.

As the authors showed in their dissection research, broad laminoarthrectomy gives access to the lateral cord if the spinal cord is carefully rotated. Through a suitable incision, a graft consisting of a fragment of a peripheral nerve can be implanted at a depth of 1 mm and secured in place with a biologic adhesive. The graft technique precludes the need for delicate, microscopically guided manipulations of obliquely angled rootlets in the tiny intradural space. Moreover, it is rare that all the rootlets in the intradural compartment are torn out in a patient with severe injury and multiple avulsions. Therefore, the length of the rootlets has no repercussions on the surgical method because the graft is long enough to cope with all eventualities.

One of the problems associated with this approach is that it is not possible to expose the surface of the ventral cord, so the graft can only be implanted in the lateral cord at a distance from the ventral root exit zone (VREZ). The other drawback is that it does not afford access to the infraclavicular brachial plexus, so that distal repair is impossible if the nerve stumps have retracted downward. Finally, it does not allow dissection of the terminal branches, which constitute a perfect means of identifying the various elements of the plexus (which is sometimes extremely difficult). Carlstedt overcame this problem by modifying the conventional posterior approach, making it more lateral so that he could perform anterior infraclavicular dissection, although he was still approaching the cord from behind.

This approach results in full exposure of the plexus from the intradural rootlets to the proximal trunks, which makes it relatively easy to evaluate the extent of the damage at the beginning of the operation. Access to the VREZ and extensive dissection of the ventral roots (as far as the spinal ganglion) make it possible to perform reimplantation in the cord of C5 through C8, because of the obliquity of the rootlet (which is particularly marked in C8). Despite the obliquity in T1, reimplantation here remains difficult. This approach is extremely invasive, however, and threatens long-term spinal stability because articular processes are removed. The dissection is long, difficult, and extremely bloody.

The current authors therefore decided to begin their clinical experimentation on rigorously selected patients with avulsion of multiple nerve roots in whom the damage already had been thoroughly evaluated before the operation.

Three patients—all injured in road accidents—were operated on between March 1999 and January 2001 in the Department of Neurosurgery of Angers University Hospital. All had a completely paralyzed arm, with total loss of sensory and motor function. The reimplantation procedure was performed 3 weeks after the accident in two of the patients, and 2 months afterward in the third patient. This time frame is relatively rapid, given the problems associated with treating this population of patients.

In each case, the posterior subscapular approach was used. The patients were placed in ventral decubitus with their head secured in a head holder at bony points to prevent lesions at the contact areas. In the first phase of the operation, the damage was thoroughly assessed, and repair was undertaken in the second phase. Complete arthrectomy and opening of the foramen were associated with the heaviest bleeding during the operation, notably from peridural veins. An understanding of the anatomy of the brachial plexus is difficult in the badly injured shoulder. The grafts were implanted at a depth of 1 mm in the lateral aspect of the cervical cord and fixed in position using a biologic adhesive. Distal connections were made using silastic tubes. The closure of the dura mater was consolidated with biologic adhesive and, if necessary, fragments of muscle tissue were removed from along the approach route. The wound was closed with a passive drain. The patients' elbows were immobilized on their bodies for 10 days during which time they wore a soft neck brace. They were then referred to a physical therapy unit for rehabilitation.

The preliminary results have not yet been published and, from a functional point of view, they are disappointing. In all three patients, however, electromyography has indicated that communications between cord and muscle have been re-established, and similarly, in all three patients, there is clear clinical evidence of muscular activity.

Of the various factors that might affect the restoration of function, the most important would seem to be the surgical method used, the nature of the original nerve root damage and any associated lesions, and the interval between the accident and surgery. In practice, recovering function depends on two main parameters: the number of surviving motor neurons in the relevant compartment of the cord and the extent of axon regrowth across the graft.

The percentage of residual motor neurons drops rapidly after the injury because neuron death occurs because of severance from the periphery and the loss of trophic substrate, a situation that is probably exacerbated by vascular ischemia [27,30]. The patients who recovered motor function were those who had been operated on early (after just 3 wk). Part of the failure is probably from technical problems during the surgical procedure, notably the difficulty in identifying distal stumps in a severely injured shoulder through a route that does not afford access to the terminal branches.

In the authors' patients, unlike those of Carlstedt, no co-contraction of opposing muscles was observed. No recovery of any sensory function was observed, including proprioception, temperature perception, or pain. This finding is not surprising because posterior roots were not repaired (except in one patient). None of the three patients, however, experienced any deafferentation pain. Can this be explained in terms of the simple reimplantation of ventral roots reestablishing the connection with the effector?

Ideal intraspinal implantation site for repairing ventral root avulsion

The risks associated with the posterior approach coupled with the poor outcomes obtained with this approach led the authors to reconsider their strategy [31]. Could the failure be from a poor choice of implantation site for the graft in the cord? The only implantation site possible with a posterior approach, even though it necessitates arthrectomy, is the white matter of the lateral cord. In the CNS, however, molecules associated with myelin and oligodendrocytes in the white matter inhibit axon regrowth [32–40]. Because it has been shown that the white matter of the cord does not permit axon regrowth, it is easy to hypothesize that inappropriate positioning of the graft in the cervical cord might explain the observed poor outcomes. Ideally, reimplantation should be performed as close as possible to the ventral horn of the gray matter.

The authors therefore undertook a microscopic study of the anatomy of the cervical cord, focusing on the five compartments into which the graft could feasibly be reimplanted. The purpose was to analyze the architecture of the ventral horn of the gray matter of the cord with respect to the ventrolateral sulcus and the arrangement and path of the motor nerve fibers that cross the white matter before arriving at the ventral root. The ultimate purpose was to identify the ideal site for reimplantation.

After traumatic avulsion of a ventral nerve root followed by reimplantation into the cervical cord, neurophysiologic data show that motor neurons are capable of projecting new axons through the reimplanted rootlets or across a peripheral nerve graft. The problem remains that implantation into white matter probably restricts axon regrowth in humans. The question was, therefore, whether a better outcome (ie, the recovery of more function) could be obtained if the reimplantation was performed near the ventral horn of the gray matter where the axonal fibers emerge. It is logical to perform reimplantation as close as possible to the cell bodies of the spinal motor neurons (ie, right next to the ventral horn).

In this regard, the ideal choice would seem to be the ventrolateral sulcus closest to the path of the avulsed axons. This study showed that the ventromedial region of the anterior horn of the gray matter represents the point of emergence of the greatest number of axons going to the ventral root across the white matter. Therefore, the site of reimplantation should be as close as possible to the ventromedial region of the anterior horn, to make the most of the orientation of the cell bodies of the motor neurons innervating the arm. This situation requires an anterior approach that affords the most ventral access possible. Ideally, the graft should be reimplanted at a depth of at least 2 mm, as vertically as possible across the ventrolateral sulcus itself (across the VREZ). Reimplantation through the ventrolateral sulcus makes it possible to avoid the spinothalamic, spinocerebellar, and the spinobulbar (ascending) tracts, and the lateral rubrospinal and reticulospinal (descending) tracts.

Therefore, the authors had to consider an anterior approach that would afford access to the cord from in front and access to an anatomic reimplantation site in the axis of the fibers across the VREZ to reach the anterior horn of the gray matter, and simultaneous access to the entire plexus, including its terminal branches.

Lateral interscalenic, multilevel, oblique corpectomies to repair ventral root avulsions after brachial plexus injury: anatomic study and first clinical experience

To allow anatomic implantation of a graft, the idea was to expose the ventral surface of the cervical medulla and the entire brachial plexus, including the subclavicular plexus, in a procedure that would not take too long, that would not destabilize the cervical spine, and that would be reproducible [41].

An interscalenic approach was chosen. This approach makes it possible from the outset to examine the extraspinal plexus and check that the interscalenic cavity is empty. It affords access to the intervertebral foramen and the ventrolateral surface of the transverse process and the vertebral body at the desired level. The bone is drilled at an oblique angle, removing half of the vertebral body without touching the joint mass (ie, not threatening stability). In the second stage, the transverse foramen may be opened, if necessary. This step mobilizes the vertebral artery (VA) and makes it possible to expose the entire intradural compartment as far as the intervertebral foramen. The main risk is injury to the sympathetic network. Dissection has shown that the implantation occurred in an anatomic situation, and allows us to confirm the reality and level of avulsions, because this approach makes it possible to visualize intact contralateral nerve roots at the same level.

Surgical anatomy of the lateral interscalenic, multilevel, oblique corpectomies

In the lateral interscalenic, multilevel, oblique corpectomy (or LIMOC approach), the anterolateral aspect of the cervical spine is approached from the injured side. The patient is placed in a supine position with his or her head in slight rotation and extension to the contralateral side. The longitudinal skin incision follows the posterior edge or medial border of the sternocleidomastoid (SCM) muscle. The incision does not extend to the tip of the mastoid, because there is no need for C2-3 exposure. The incision, however, may extend to the suprasternal notch to expose the C7-T1 level and to the deltopectoralis sulcus along the caudal edge of the clavicle for an infraclavicular dissection. Sharp dissection passes behind the deep aspect of the SCM muscle, which is retracted anteriorly and medially. The accessory nerve does not need to be identified because the C3-4 level was not being exposed. Using the approach, the great vessels, trachea, and esophagus are left undissected and protected by the SCM muscle. The cervical spine is then approached between the scalene muscles by following the cervical nerve roots. The transverse processes can be identified by touch and are covered by the prevertebral muscle mass. Control and freeing of the phrenic nerve are mandatory before resection of the anterior scalene muscle at its insertion level on the tubercules of the transverse processes, because the nerve runs under the muscle's aponeurosis. Starting from the tip of the transverse processes, both the aponeurosis of the longus colli muscle and the sympathetic chain are then retracted medially. Small rami communicantes are necessarily sacrificed on the chosen levels. Care must be taken to avoid injury of the VA if it runs in front of the transverse processes. Preoperative angiography is important to ascertain whether the VA enters the transverse canal at a typical level. At this point, all of the transverse processes and the lateral aspect of the vertebral bodies at the desired levels are exposed. The intertransversarii muscles and bone overlying the VA must be carefully resected, taking care to preserve the periosteal sheath surrounding VA and venous plexus. Once this is completed, the periosteal sheath is opened under magnification along the desired length, so that the VA can be completely mobilized. The drilling of the remaining transverse processes is then started and extended obliquely through the vertebral bodies. The anterolateral dura, entire spinal nerve roots, and supraclavicular plexus are exposed. The dura is opened longitudinally along with the separate dural layers of each spinal nerve root. Contralateral ventral rootlets, ipsilateral location of the VREZs, and anterior spinal artery and anastomoses are identified. The use of an endoscope allows the surgeon to make a diagnosis of avulsion along the entire length of the cervical cord.

The direct implantation of avulsed roots or of a sural nerve graft through the VREZ itself is easy. The implant should be positioned 2 mm deep to the pia matter, and parallel to the ventral sulcus of the cord, using a myringotome. In doing so, the surgeon may reach the ventromedial aspect of the ventral gray horn, as previously shown by the current authors' works. Two or three grafts can be performed, depending on the surgical plan and the clinical condition of the patient. For long grafts, there is no need for vertebral artery mobilization, and the grafts run in front of the artery and phrenic nerve. Collagen or silastic tubes are easily placed at the distal stump, if necessary. The dura is closed with sutures, which are reinforced using fibrin glue and muscle. No fusion is necessary, even if LIMOC is performed on many levels.

This anatomic analysis made it possible for the authors to begin their clinical experimentation and perform implantation in their first four patients. These four patients are the first—and so far the only—patients on whom this novel technique has been practiced. The results are promising, but evaluation is still underway.

This technique should allow the surgeon to perform reimplantation by means of a peripheral nerve graft in an ideal anatomic position across the VREZ itself, at the same time repairing any distal lesions of the plexus that are in evidence. The method is not excessively invasive. It does not take an inordinate amount of time nor does it entail arthrodesis. With the authors' experience and after analysis of the first results, this surgical technique might prove to be a modality of choice for the repair of nerve root avulsion.

It is as yet too early to perform a serious analysis of outcomes because the first operation was performed only 18 months ago. Nevertheless, it is already possible to make certain observations.

The first concerns the long intervals between injury and surgery in all four of these patients— between 4 and 8 months. After this length of time, the general level of muscular atrophy is marked and the number of residual motor neurons in the anterior horn low. Therefore, the conditions for these trial operations were poor, although this situation is common in such patients who often have multiple injuries so that the damage to the brachial plexus goes unnoticed for a long time. All the work done previously—in both humans and animals—has shown the importance of operating as early as possible [27,42].

The second observation concerns the seriousness of the lesions. None of the patients had any identifiable nerve stumps in the interscalenic cavity, so to reach the subclavicular plexus, the authors had to use grafts that were probably too long. The length and number of grafts are limited, and caliber is often a problem. It is unclear whether the small number of axons would be capable of regenerating over a significant length across the graft (ie, how many would be capable of re-creating a functional motor end plate in an atrophied muscle).

Despite these adverse circumstances and the fact that no more than 18 months have elapsed since the first operation, three of four of these patients are presenting clear signs that communication has been re-established between spinal cord and muscle, with evidence of muscle activity.

It is difficult to say to what extent the observed recovery is specific to the surgical reimplantation. Collateral or aberrant regeneration can result in recovery. Specific neurons can only be identified by means of the methods of intracellular physiology or histologic analysis, neither of which is possible in humans. Therefore, there is no absolute proof to show that specific regeneration has occurred directly from the authors' intervention. This problem led them to choose, in certain patients, a graft directly connected to the terminal branch of the plexus. The results are important and indicate that reimplantation is playing a role in the recovery. Similarly, the authors have not combined nerve root reimplantation with conventional neurotization methods to avoid complicating the results. It is clear that such combination therapy might be useful in the future, once the authors' method has been definitively evaluated.

Two surgical limitations were quickly evident. First, oblique somatotomy targets the roots to be reimplanted and an exhaustive examination of the damage as a whole is therefore not possible. Perioperative radiographic examination during the operation identifies which vertebrae—and therefore which roots—are affected but uncertainty remains about the ventral roots above and below, and even about the dorsal roots. This problem could be overcome by using a flexible endoscope inside the spinal canal, similar to Carlstedt's method. Second, dorsal roots cannot be reimplanted by means of this approach. Recovering some degree of proprioception is important and necessary for useful muscle function, however, not so much for the control of simple movements (eg, flexion and extension of the elbow or abduction of the shoulder) but rather for fine movements, such as the contraction of hand muscles. This aspect warrants consideration.

Perspectives

Reimplantation surgery of the brachial plexus: the place of neurotrophic factors

With this surgical method, several questions remain unanswered and certain limitations have become clear, notably the fact that a long interval between the injury and the operation is bound to curtail the degree of recovery possible.

It was long believed that differentiated neurons could not regenerate in the adult CNS. As previously discussed, physicians now know that this capacity exists, although in the real world its power is limited.

The problem of glial healing and inhibitory substances in the white matter can be overcome by performing implantation in the cord near the ventral horn of the gray matter rather than directly in the white matter. Schwann cells from the peripheral graft are probably not able to produce the key neurotrophic factors in sufficient quantity to compensate for the local deficiency of these key mediators, so the aim must be to provide them directly in situ.

A group working at the Mayo Clinic recently conducted a review of the literature concerning the manufacture and use of biodegradable polymers in implants for the treatment of spinal cord injuries [43]. The microarchitecture of these implants includes two parallel channels that are designed to reproduce the long channels of the medulla and that could guide axon regrowth. Such regrowth might be further stimulated if neurotrophic factors or genetically modified Schwann cells were incorporated into these implants. The problem remains as to whether such implants (which have a diameter of 3 mm and are 5 mm long) can be introduced into injured spinal cord tissue without exacerbating the damage. The bulk of these implants means that they cannot be used in healthy cord where multiple avulsion has occurred; these implants therefore do not represent a practical option in their present configuration.

Alternatively, can neurotrophic factors be applied parallel to spinal repair of avulsion? This method would necessitate targeting and in situ administration because of the following factors:

1. Neurotrophic factors are labile species with very short biologic half-lives, and they cannot cross the blood-brain barrier if they are administered systemically.
2. Side effects in the periphery are always observed because receptors for the various neurotrophic factors are so widely distributed throughout the body.
3. The activities of neurotrophic factors are spatially defined in the CNS.

Therefore, if any of these factors is to be exploited, it will be necessary to have it available in the kind of pharmaceutical presentation that ensures that the compound will be active in the target tissue. Several different strategies have been developed. The controlled release from cells (eg, fibroblasts or Schwann cells) that have been genetically modified to produce a neurotrophic factor is not yet a viable option [44], but the use of loaded biodegradable microspheres has been perfected in Angers [45–47]. A method based on the encapsulation of an active substance is in routine use in our neurosurgery department in the treatment of malignant subtentorial glioma in adults. This type of system has several advantages, including protection of the active species, control of the quantity administered and the rate of administration over a longer or shorter time frame, and accurate targeting of the region to be treated. The caliber of the microspheres means that they can be administered by injection.

The first stage of the project is to investigate the efficacy of neurotrophic supplementation in animal models of nerve root avulsion, with the neurotrophic factors administered in the form of biodegradable microspheres injected directly into the spinal parenchyma. The authors hope to show that this strategy contributes significantly to maintaining neuron numbers if reimplantation is performed either immediately after avulsion or 3 weeks later. One endpoint to be studied will be the recovery of motor function. Extensive animal experiments will be performed before attempting to transfer the technology into humans.

Summary

Currently, the authors' research confirms that, in humans, communication between the cord and effector muscles can be re-established after multiple nerve root avulsion by the implantation of peripheral nerve grafts. Outcomes are still modest, but the possibility of improvement exists. The technique of reimplantation makes it possible to envisage global repair with the possibility of repair of all avulsed regions. The most important factor that could maximize the extent of functional recovery is reducing the time between the injury and corrective surgery: the diagnosis of avulsion within 10 days and reparative surgery within 3 weeks is the objective. This goal will involve a global re-evaluation of how these patients are managed. The problem of the recovery of sensory function (tactile and fine perception and proprioception) warrants further work.

It seems likely that methods combining medullary reimplantation with neurotization will be the best way of correcting these lesions of the brachial plexus. In this context, cross-disciplinary collaboration is probably more important than ever. The place that methods based on reimplantation will have in the final picture remains to be seen. The key question is in which patients should medullary reimplantation be attempted and which method should be used. Moreover, medullary reimplantation should be considered as an adjunct to all other surgical options and should not compromise the chance of the latter modalities to be effective.

An important point remains: are physicians going to be able to map out all the boundaries of this question in the future?

References

[1] Narakas AO. Thoughts on neurotization or nerve transfers in irreparable nerve lesions. Clin Plast Surg 1984;11:153–60.
[2] Ovelmen-Levitt J. Abnormal physiology of the dorsal horn as related to the deafferentation syndrome. Appl Neurophysiol 1988;51:104–16.
[3] Asfadourian H, Tramond B, Dauge MC, Oberlin C. Morphometric study of the upper intercostals nerves: practical application for neurotizations in traumatic brachial plexus palsies [in French]. Chir Main 1999;18(4):243–53.
[4] Loy S, Bhatia A, Asfadourian H, Oberlin C. Ulnar nerve fascicle transfer onto to the biceps muscle nerve in C5–C6 or C5–C6-C7 avulsions of the brachial plexus. Eighteen cases [in French]. Ann Chir Main Memb Super 1997;16(4):275–84.
[5] Oberlin C, Beal D, Leechavengvongs S, Salon A, Dauge MC, Sarcy JJ. Nerve transfer to biceps muscle using a part of ulnar nerve for C5–C6 avulsion of the brachial plexus: anatomical study and report of four cases. J Hand Surg [Am] 1994;19(2):232–7.
[6] Aguayo AJ, David S, Bray GM. Influences of the glial environment on the elongation of axons after injury: transplantation studies in adult rodents. J Exp Biol 1981;95:231–40.
[7] Aguayo AJ, David S, Richardson P, Bray GM. Axonal regeneration in peripheral and central nervous system transplants. Adv Cell Neurobiol 1982;3: 215–34.
[8] David S, Aguayo AJ. Axonal elongation into peripheral nervous system "bridges" after central nervous system injury in adult rats. Science 1981; 214:933–5.
[9] Richardson PM, Issa VM, Aguayo AJ. Regeneration of long spinal axons in the rat. J Neurocytol 1984;13(1):165–82.
[10] Richardson PM, McGuiness UM, Aguayo AJ. Peripheral nerve autografts to the rat spinal cord: studies with axonal tracing methods. Brain Res 1982;237(1):147–62.
[11] Chai H, Wu W, So KF, Yip HK. Survival and regeneration of motoneurons in adult rats by reimplantation of ventral root following spinal root avulsion. Neuroreport 2000;11(6):1249–52.
[12] Acheson A, Barker PA, Alderson RF, Miller FD, Murphy RA. Detection of brain-derived neurotrophic factor-like activity in fibroblasts and Schwann

cells: inhibition by antibodies to NGF. Neuron 1991; 7:265–75.

[13] Bixby JL, Lilien J, Reichardt LF. Identification of the major proteins that promote neuronal outgrowth on Schwann cells in vitro. J Cell Biol 1988; 107:353–61.

[14] Bunge MB. Schwann cell regulation of extracellular matrix biosynthesis and assembly. In: Dyck PJ, Thomas PK, Griffin JW, Low PA, Poduslo JF, editors. Peripheral neuropathy. Philadelphia: WB Saunders; 1993. p. 299–316.

[15] Davis GE, Manthorpe M, Varon S. Parameters of neuritic growth from ciliary ganglion neurons in vitro: influence of laminin, schwannoma polyorithine-binding neurite promoting factor and ciliary neurotrophic factor. Brain Res 1985;349(1–2): 75–84.

[16] Fernandez E, Pallini R, Mercanti D. Effects of topically administered nerve growth factor on axonal regeneration in peripheral nerve autografts implanted in the spinal cord of rats. Neurosurgery 1990;26:37–42.

[17] Friedman B, Scherer SS, Rudge JS, et al. Regulation of ciliary neurotrophic factor expression in myelin-related Schwann cells in vivo. Neuron 1992;9: 295–305.

[18] Heumann R, Korsching S, Bandtlow C, Thoenen H. Changes of nerve growth factor synthesis in non-neuronal cells in response to sciatic nerve transection. J Cell Biol 1887;104:1623–31.

[19] Kleinmann HK, Kleber RJ, Martin GR. Role of collagenous matrices in the adhesion and growth of cells. J Cell Biol 1981;88:473–85.

[20] Martini R. Expression and functional roles of neural cell surface molecules and extracellular matrix components during development and regeneration of peripheral nerves. J Neurocytol 1994;23:1–28.

[21] Meyer M, Matsuoka I, Wetmore C, Olson L, Thoenen H. Enhanced synthesis of brain-derived neurotrophic factor in the lesioned peripheral nerve. Different mechanisms are responsible for the regulation of BDNF and NGF mRNA. J Cell Biol 1992; 119:45–54.

[22] Rende M, Muir D, Ruoslahti E, Hagg T, Varon S, Manthorpe M. Immunolocalization of ciliary neurotrophic factor in adult rat sciatic nerve. Glia 1992;5: 25–32.

[23] Schachner M. Functional implications of glial cell recognition molecules. Semin Neurosci 1990;2: 497–507.

[24] Frazier CH, Skillern PG. Supraclavicular subcutaneous lesions of the brachial plexus not associated with skeletal injuries. JAMA 1911;57:1957–63.

[25] Bonney G, Jamieson A. Reimplantation of C7 and C8. Communication au symposium sur le plexus brachial. Int Microsurg 1979;1:103–6.

[26] Carlstedt T, Grane P, Hallin RG, Noren G. Return of function after spinal cord implantation of avulsed spinal nerve root. Lancet 1995;346:1323–5.

[27] Carlstedt T, Anand P, Hallin R, Misra PV, Noren G, Seferlis T. Spinal nerve root repair and reimplantation of avulsed ventral roots into the spinal cord after brachial plexus injury. J Neurosurg 2000;93: 237–47.

[28] Fournier HD, Mercier P, Menei P. Anatomical bases of the posterior approach to the brachial plexus for repairing avulsed spinal nerve roots. Surg Radiol Anat 2001;23:3–8.

[29] Kline DG, Kott J, Barnes G, Bryant L. Exploration of selected brachial plexus lesions by the posterior subscapular approach. J Neurosurg 1978;49: 872–80.

[30] Birch R, Bonney G, Wynn Parry CB. Surgical disorders of the peripheral nerves. London: Churchill Livingston; 1998.

[31] Fournier HD, Menei P, Khalifa R, Mercier P. Ideal intraspinal implantation site for the repair of ventral root avulsion after brachial plexus injury in humans. A preliminary anatomical study. Surg Radiol Anat 2001;23:191–5.

[32] Schwab ME. Molecules inhibiting neurite growth: a minireview. Neurochem Res 1996;21:755–61.

[33] Schwab ME. Structural plasticity of the adult CNS. Negative control by neurite growth inhibitory signals. Int J Dev Neurosci 1996;14:379–85.

[34] Schwab ME, Kapfhammer JP, Bandtlow CE. Inhibitors of neurite growth. Annu Rev Neurosci 1993;16: 565–95.

[35] Schwab ME. Experimental aspects of spinal cord regeneration. Curr Opin Neurol Neurosurg 1993; 6(4):549–53.

[36] Schwab ME, Caroni P. Oligodendrocytes and CNS myelin are nonpermissive substrates for neurite growth and fibroblast spreading in vitro. J Neurosci 1991;11:2381–93.

[37] Schwab ME. Myelin-associated inhibitors of neurite growth. Exp Neurol 1990;109:2–5.

[38] Thallmair M, Metz GAS, Graggen WJZ, Raineteau O, Kartje GL, Schwab ME. Neurite growth inhibitors restrict plasticity and functional recovery following corticospinal tract lesions. Nat Neurosci 1998;1:124–31.

[39] Pot C, Simonen M, Weinmann O, et al. Nogo-A expressed in Schwann cells impairs axonal regeneration after peripheral nerve injury. J Cell Biol 2002; 159(1):29–35.

[40] Taketomi M, Kinoshita N, Kimura K, et al. Nogo-A expression in mature oligodendrocytes of rat spinal cord in association with specific molecules. Neurosci Lett 2002;332(1):37.

[41] Fournier HD, Mercier P, Menei P. Lateral interscalenic multilevel oblique corpectomies to repair ventral root avulsions after brachial plexus injury in humans: anatomical study and first clinical experience. J Neurosurg 2001;95:202–7.

[42] Holtzer CA, Feirabend HK, Marani E, Thomeer RT. Ultrastructural and quantitative motoneuronal changes after ventral root avulsion favor early

surgical repair. Arch Physiol Biochem 2000;108(3):
293–309.

[43] Friedman JA, Windebank AJ, Moore MJ, Spinner
RJ, Currier BL, Yaszemski MJ. Biodegradable poly-
mer grafts for surgical repair of the injured spinal
cord. Neurosurgery 2002;51(3):742–52.

[44] Menei P, Montero-Menei C, Whittemore SR, Bunge
RP, Bunge MB. Schwann cells genetically modified
to secrete human BDNF promote enhanced axonal
regrowth across transected rat spinal cord. Eur J
Neurosci 1998;10:607–21.

[45] Benoit JP, Faisant N, Venier-Julienne MC, Menei P.
Development of microspheres for neurological dis-

orders: from basics to clinical applications. J Control
Release 2000;65(1–2):285–96.

[46] Pean JM, Venier-Julienne MC, Boury F, Menei P,
Denizot B, Benoit JP. NGF release from poly (d,
I-lactide-co-glycolide) microspheres. Effect of
some formulation parameters on encapsulated
NGF stability. J Controlled Release 1998;56:
175–87.

[47] Gouhier C, Chalon S, Aubert-Pouessel A, et al.
Protection of dopaminergic nigrostriatal afferents
by GDNF delivered by microspheres in a rodent
model of Parkinson's disease. Synapse 2002;44:
124–31.

ELSEVIER
SAUNDERS

Hand Clin 21 (2005) 119–121

HAND
CLINICS

Index

Note: Page numbers of article titles are in **boldface** type.

Changing Your Address?

Make sure your subscription changes too! When you notify us of your new address, you can help make our job easier by including an exact copy of your Clinics label number with your old address (see illustration below.) This number identifies you to our computer system and will speed the processing of your address change. Please be sure this label number accompanies your old address and your corrected address—you can send an old Clinics label with your number on it or just copy it exactly and send it to the address listed below.

We appreciate your help in our attempt to give you continuous coverage. Thank you.

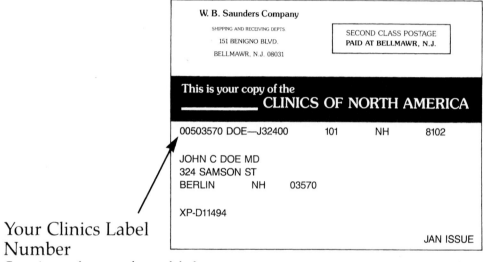

Your Clinics Label Number
Copy it exactly or send your label
along with your address to:
W.B. Saunders Company, Customer Service
Orlando, FL 32887-4800
Call Toll Free 1-800-654-2452

Please allow four to six weeks for delivery of new subscriptions and for processing address changes.